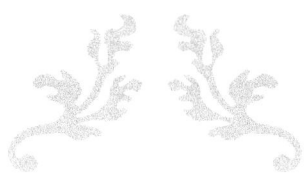

CREATING THE DYNAMIC DEMENTIA CARE TEAM- REVISED

By Clarice Cagle Cook

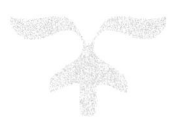

Copyright

This manual contains skill information for self-evaluation, brain anatomy of persons with dementia and how to interact, communicate, and help provide quality of life for those with brain related deficits and/or dementia.

Dedication

I am so grateful and blessed.

I wish to give credit for training and advice to the Alzheimer's Association, to my care giving and disability employers, teachers, trainers, college professors, clients and fellow caregivers who have all been instrumental in my development as a writer and caregiver.

There is no way that I can thank my ancestors, aunts, grandmothers, and mother from whom I received the care giving markers and desire to help others. They are all gone now, but as long as they are not forgotten, their legacy will live on through those left behind.

Thank you to my extraordinary husband who has found other things to do while I spend hours in caregiving and sitting behind the computer. I've been in training to take care of him someday. I sincerely hope he doesn't have to take care of me.

I appreciate all my dance instructors who taught me to dance, because dancing has kept me younger. Hopefully, the dance will not end too soon. I have a lot more to do.

Most of all, I am so grateful for all my dementia care clients and to my step dad of thirty-four years, William Robert Howe. He was there for me in so many difficult situations. I so wish that I had been able to help him with the difficult journey in more educated and profound ways. Because of him, I have been more focused on memory loss and those who have joined him in this fight. Thank you, Dad.

Please support your local Alzheimer's Association, which also reaches out to and supports other dementia diseases. Go to Alz.org to find out ways to volunteer, walk for, and donate for research in finding cure for increasing and devastating memory loss diseases that can start in the 40's and earlier.

Message to the Caregiver

This manual is intended to inform, excite, enhance, and add to the experience of family and professional caregivers. You will find repeat information throughout to show correlation and o emphasize the different reasons for the importance of methods of communication and interaction. Readers are encouraged to use the contents for reference, to enhance learned methods, and to learn new techniques. Throughout the book, there are quizzes. Taking notes and self-testing are recommended. Reviews are appreciated.

Before and during reading and going through the exercises in this manual, it would serve the professional or family caregiver, potential or active; to access self-identity. It is important to you in life.

In order to be able to deal with another person's life you must be able to value yourself and take care of your own body and soul. Doing so will bring you an open mind uncluttered by what other people think of you. You will have the confidence you need to perform and interact in some very difficult situations.

From birth, every individual has unique markers in the brain that determine ability to react to the circumstances in life. However, events, how people treat us, whom we meet, and how we interpret daily life information sets up our values as we mentally and emotionally grow into who we are.

Evaluate Self Honestly
At the end of this manual is a guide to evaluation. It is recommended that caregivers take this opportunity for self-examination after reading through all the chapters.

Do you take care of others because everyone else says you are "good at it" or that it is a job and you need it for financial reasons? If that is the case, assess yourself and find out what it is that truly inspires you. Caregiving does not pay all that well monetarily and time is more valuable than money.

To be an effective caregiver, you must have a passion for it and be able to take care of self-needs. Otherwise, you will be thinking about ways that you can survive the shift, or get out of the shift. You will find yourself in conflict with family, friends and the agency or the client's family.

I cannot emphasize it enough. Therefore, I am repeating the above in a more definite way. Identifying yourself as a caregiver means that you have to put a value on the time and effort for a day's work. However, if you are embarking on a career as a professional caregiver solely because you need the money, it is time for you to find out whom you are. Accepting how other people define you is asking for an eventual burn and crash. It is not fair to you or your client to muddle through or fight against what is natural to you and your purpose in life.

Suggested reading: Dr. Phil McGraw's Authentic Self and Stedman Graham's Identity: Your Process for Success.

About the Author
In order to give understanding about what it takes to be a caregiver, I think it might help to listen to others who have taken that journey. The following is my story.

As a certified nurse aide in the 1990's, I worked in a nursing home. At that time, in-home caregivers were unheard of. When I went into the on-the-job training for my certification, I was at the bottom of the economical chain and had no place to go but up. My main incentive was to survive. It was not that I did not care about people. I knew that I had the compassion, but I had no idea who I was inside out. I absorbed and believed what everyone else said about me. I really did not like myself at all, but I felt obligated to find a way to support myself to keep from being a burden on others.

As it turned out, the patients taught me about the meaning of life, and without realizing it, a crusty old head nurse made me face reality. When she saw me shedding tears in the hall, after I had been listening to anguish of a patient, she said, "Clarice, you need to get out of this business if you can't control your emotions." I had an ah ha moment. I then felt the fruitless ness of trying to make a difference in a nursing home in a time where people went to die and indeed in those days even more than now, wanted to die. I couldn't realize then that I was making a difference to each of those people with a moment by moment connection. It meant a lot to each of them to have someone with a smile to make their last days important and to care. However, quality of life was not the atmosphere created by the nursing home profession of that day.

I went home that night with a plan. I wanted to help people to live in the moment with quality of life, not live every day looking forward at death.

The next day, I applied at a local disability workshop. I got a job as a work service instructor helping people with disabilities find quality of life in society. I was making a difference. I started to learn about humility, and how to think and live from the inside out.

I was already taking psychology and self-help classes in the community college and now I was learning on the job how to assess myself and gain the confidence I needed to help others. I also learned that keeping vigilant and continuing to learn about others and self was and will always be a continuing lifetime commitment.

Life was no longer something I took for granted, and I started to wake every morning with purpose to help others outside my family and myself. I had raised my daughters to be self-sufficient while fulfilling my purpose.

Moving to a college town, I changed to a four-year institution. I worked in business during my late blooming, growing up years. Since I could only get financial help by taking in business classes, I obtained a business degree with honors.

To try to satisfy my need to write, I wrote and published two tabloid type magazines. This had me scattered, but I balanced my need with my passions as best I could.

In assessing myself during those years, I continually ask myself questions and did a lot of journaling about how I felt about what I was doing. As it turned out, I went at everything I did with passion. However, I was most passionate (and still am) in helping others, learning from others, showing others what I have learned, and writing.

With age, I lost what perceived youthful physical beauty I had, but gained reality that came from within. I was no longer what everyone else thought I should be or may still think that I should be. Today, I balance my need for financial security, writing, and care giving.

The business degree that I earned came out of necessity, because that was the only way that I could get the scholarships and grants to go to college, but I did and do love business, and it has helped me in my end goals.

I think I have found myself and that I am fulfilling my purpose as a dementia care practitioner, activities and memory caregiver, writer and teacher. It is all coming together because I am in control of my destiny, while recognizing myself for who I am and practicing my own values.

One of my greatest moments came when I started to understand the brain and how it works. Understanding the process of the programming that goes on from babyhood, helped me to forgive myself for the mistakes I have made and to be able to forgive others. It all starts to make sense and helps us in our communication skills with others when we know that we are who we are because of what we've been taught, what others expect us to be and what events and concepts we've allowed to affect us and form our persona. Most of all, I learned not to have unreasonable expectations.

NOTES

Chapter One -Taking Care of the Caregiver

This is a personal note to both professional and family caregivers. It is not a lecture. It is a discussion to those who put everyone ahead of himself or herself. Eventually they find that they have nothing else left to give. This chapter provides information on where to look for help and gives tips that others have used to keep a mental and physical balance for self while caring for others.

In my experience in the work field, I have noticed big mistakes in others and myself that have led to stumbles and sometimes failure.

Number 1: Do not be closed to learning from others, from the experts, from co-workers, from the families and from the person with dementia. Not even the scientists know it all.

Number 2: Be a team member. Allow and acknowledge mistakes in others and most of all self.

Number 3: When approaching others about mistakes or your perspective, remember respect. "I have a suggestion," or "Sometimes it works best for me if..."

Number 4: Respect self and go forward with positive solutions for the future. Mistakes are great opportunities to learn.

Dedicated caregivers are prone to neglect themselves, forgetting that they too have a human brain and body that needs love and nurturing. Without good health, the body and brain breaks down and the caregiver may face more illness and other problems. The ability to care for others begins to take a toll.

Since the brain relies on the health of the body and the body relies on the health of the brain, sleep, good nutrition, exercise, good health care, and stress reduction are all essential.

Medical experts have determined that while everyone is different in many ways, there are basic health care steps that everyone can take to protect themselves. Some requirements are more difficult for caregivers to achieve; however, it can be done.

The caregiver starts by keeping a journal, setting up a self-care and health care plan, keeping doctor and dental appointments and paying attention to and participating in exercise and nutritional need activities. Sleep should also be on the top of the list.

By the end of the last paragraph, I can mentally hear the chuckling and clucking coming from other caregivers, especially the last sentence. "Sleep...do you mean sleep walking?"

Sleep Deprivation
For those who work night shifts, this may or may not be a problem. Some caregivers have said they love the night shift. Others walk around like zombies and struggle to stay awake throughout the night.

Professional caregivers should never work the night shift if they cannot obtain sufficient sleep during daytime hours...period. Staying alert is why you were hired to be in the home of a client or to attend needs of more than one in a group setting. Hospitals who hire sitters for patients who are a falling risk or need companionship for one reason or the other will fire a caregiver who closes their eyes for a rest.

There is an old myth that states that everyone has different requirements for sleep and that some can be alert with four hours while others need ten hours. This may be half-truth. The truth is that people who only get four hours' sleep are most likely running on caffeine, or other additive to their body, or sleep walking. They may only think they are operating at full capacity.

A brain and body that is running like an engine for twenty hours and is only idle for four hours will not be able to function as well as a brain and body that is running for fourteen hours and is idle for ten hours.

Lack of sleep is the culprit of many mistakes. The brain needs idle time to process information, put to rest troubles, give the mind peace, and give the other important organs of the body rest. A troubled mind at bedtime may deter the brain from relaxing and going into idle mode or stress from the events of the day might render troubled sleep.

Sleeping pills only make a person relax enough to be asleep; however, research shows that sleep from drugs does not truly put the brain into a restful sleep. People are still tired throughout the following wake hours.

People who have a hard time staying asleep at night, have restless sleep and other deterrents to getting a good eight to ten hours of sleep should consult their health care providers for solutions. Sleep Apnea, restless leg syndrome and other causes may be culprits and health care professionals can diagnose, treat, and help find solutions to sleep deprivation.

Nutrition Burn
It has taken many years for many health care professionals to admit that more than chemicals and just plain eating three meals a day is sufficient for good health. It is now established that nutrition with balanced meals and evaluation of individual nutrition needs is important in treating many diseases and maintaining good health.

The difficulty is that everyone has different needs. Each person needs to evaluate what is lacking and what is unnecessary for his or her own body and brain.

There is a lot of good online information now that can help with individualized nutrition and exercise plans. Some gyms offer BMI (Body Mass Index) and BMR (Basal Metabolic Rate). Body Mass Index measures the rate of fat to muscle in the body. Basal Metabolic Rate measures the rate that calories, fat and nutrition is burned in digestion.

In evaluating self for the health care profession, think first love of the job and then money. There is no fair monetary compensation for care giving.

In planning meals for the client/loved one, think about the caregiver nutrition needs. Clients eat better if the meal time is shared with someone else. It is a good time to lift spirits and share the day.

Quiz –Taking Care of the Caregiver

Susie has been finding herself lethargic and tired. She finds it hard to stay alert, pleasant, and attentive in caring for her clients. What of the following reasons might apply to Susan's lack of effective care giving?

A. Susie gets up very early in the morning to care for her family, runs errands and does her own housekeeping, or works all day and then all night. She rarely or never gets eight full hours of restful sleep. Sometimes she takes sleep aides which results in hyperactivity.
B. Susie wakes frequently during the night and is often anxious or depressed, snores and thrashes about the bed. She wakes in the morning tired and requires caffeine or other stimulants to get her going. The doctor suggests she might have sleep apnea.
C. Susie eats on the run and rarely has time to eat a balanced meal, chewing slowly. She eats a lot of junk food and high sugar sodas.
D. Susie never has time for structured exercise that brings up the heart rate, enhances oxygen and blood flow to the brain, relieves stress, and keeps the immune system stimulated.
E. Susie is overweight and is bored with any kind of exercise. She has no energy to do anything but lie down and sleep when she is relaxed. She has a hard time keeping awake and often falls asleep when caring for her clients.
F. All of the above.

 Recommended reading: At Alz.com – An article by Clarice Cook, Caring for the Caregiver Health Tips to Relieve Stress

Chapter Two - BRAIN INTERACTION

The Information Pathway

Excerpts and new information from caregiver articles published in Examiner.com, by Clarice Cook.

Caregiver Responsibility
Caregivers should not try to diagnose diseases or disorders. However, having a good understanding of what is happening in the brain of the client or loved one is helpful in being able to communicate and interact with that person.

There are a great many dementia disorders. Irreversible types, such as, Alzheimer's, Lewy Body and Vascular Dementia are the most diagnosed and are sometimes closely related in symptoms. All dementias are an indication of brain damage in parts of the brain.

It is the caregiver's responsibility to understand that learning and recall is impossible in the damaged areas. However, never assume that someone cannot learn or recall in the remaining viable areas. In irreversible dementia, the disease will move on to claim the entire brain. In some cases, symptoms may fluctuate, indicating beginning deterioration in that area (neurons sometimes sparking and at other times not).

Caregivers are responsible to log these symptoms as they occur with event, date, and time in order to alert change in the disease to the health care professionals and family. If the caregiver works for an agency, some more serious incidents should be reported directly and verbally when they happen. This advice is the same for any client or loved one.

What is Happening?
The greatest scientists do not know all of what is happening in the brain of someone with memory loss, because every person is different in many ways. However, researchers have determined the basic information such as processing, storage, recall, hormonal and chemical components.

Scientific research has also found what can go wrong and has identified the many diseases and disorders of dementia. With all that information, therapeutic treatment is available to alleviate the symptoms.

It helps to envision the brain as a computer system. The nervous system in the brain is like the electrical impulses and the memory chips in the motherboard and other storage and ports where data is collected and stored.

Arteries and blood vessels are responsible for delivery of nutrients and oxygen to the entire brain system. In this way, the brain can be compared to an engine. Nothing works without gas and oil. Nothing works well without a clean filter in the breather. In other words, the brain cannot work without oxygen and nutrition, and this is what happens if the arteries and veins are clogged.

The Cerebrum is the computer main frame.
The main part of the brain (thinking area) is called the Cerebrum. Within the Cerebrum are the sections that remember, solve problems, and create thought, movement, and feelings when touched. Different actions and memories are processed in separate areas or lobes within the Cerebrum.

The brain is filled with arteries that lead to veins and capillaries. This network nourishes the neurons, the nerve cells, and the memory 'chips'. Therefore, there must be the right nutrition intake in order to keep the thinking, processing, problem solving, motor movements and touch sensory functioning correctly.

Exercising the body and the brain keeps the blood pumping nutrition and oxygen throughout the neuron network to bring about balance to the electrical system.

The Cortex is the wrinkled outer layer of the Cerebrum.
Each area of the Cortex takes care of certain functions. These functions happen in the approximately 100 billion nerve cells with connections that scientist called the "neuron forest." The brain cells, (the neurons or nerve cells) are where "tangles" occur causing dementia such as Alzheimer's disease.

The Central Nervous System
The center areas of the brain (Diencephalons) carry the central nervous pathways, the Thalamus, Hypothalamus, and Epithalamiums back and forth through the Cerebral Hemispheres.

The Thalamus processes all incoming impulses from most sensory pathways. The broad connections are to movement (motor skills) for action and reaction, senses (visual, sound, and association) to regulate awareness, and integrates sensory emotional responses, such as crying or laughing.

The Thalamus sends on the responses to the hypothalamus that is concerned with automatic emotional behavior, regulation of the nervous system that controls the involuntary and related physical functioning of the body, (breathing, heartbeat, etc.), autonomic reflexes with emotional reactions, and activation of the drive to hunger and the satisfaction or satiety following the fulfillment of that drive.

The hypothalamus, located on either side of the inner brain maintains neural connections to lobes of the brain cortex, which is discussed in chapter three, "Overall Brain Function and Nervous System Interaction" and chapter four, "The Cerebral Cortex, The Thinking Wrinkles." These nuclear masses connect with the Frontal and Temporal lobes, and brain stem and a nerve mass called the Neurohypophysis with its hormones (Neurosecretions).

The Epithalamium is the pineal gland, the only unpaired structure in the brain. It produces melatonin (a pigment producing hormone) in a synthesis that controls the "body clock," (sleep rhythm, day time activity). Night opposed to day functions are influenced by the Epithalamiums. Scientists believe that the Epithalamiums may have connections to onset of puberty and ovarian/testicular activity.

Neurons and Synapses
Within the gray matter and white masses of the brain are the pathways (nerve cells and neuro-transmitters) that interact to create action and communicate to start the interaction of stored memory.

Imagine a round cell (neuron) with 'ventricles' (synapses) shooting out from all around the sphere. These ventricles lead out and at the end are 'limbs' much like a tree trunk with branches.

Within the neurons and synapses are 'wires' or 'strands' that carry the information along the paths. At the end of the 'limbs' (neuro-transmitters), the information shoots out or 'sparks' to other neuro-transmitters that send the information on further down the paths. The information normally happens in a split second and there are millions of these nerve cell clusters in the brain.

Neurons (brain cells) carry and store information.
Tracks in the nerve cells are the transport system for important nutrients and other elements and for the data that enters through the senses.

According to reports of autopsies performed on people who have died from Alzheimer's, the insides of neurons show that the pathways are excessively phosphorylated with the tau protein. Tau protein normally helps the tracks in nerve cells stay straight. Tau protein is naturally modified with phosphate molecules. However, if there is an excessive amount of phosphorylation, neuro-fibrillary tangles form and the tau collapse. The neuron transport tracks fall apart and disintegrate.

The Synapse is the connection between the nerve cells.
In a diseased brain, the connections or Synapse between the neurons are clumped together into sticky plagues of protein pieces called beta-amyloid.

According to Alz.org, scientists believe that the small clumps of beta-amyloid may block the cell-to-cell signaling at synapses and activate immune system cells that trigger inflammation and devour disabled cells. This leaves a void and if new cells do not develop memory, brain functioning loses that link. The brain area can no longer be fed; therefore, the cell dies.

The process of the dying neurons spreads through the brain. Typically, Alzheimer's can start twenty years before discovery is made. The mild stages can last two to ten years and the severe cases can last from one to five years. For many, the disease is called the long good bye.

Arteries and Blood Vessels

Anatomy terms for the blood and oxygen pathways to and throughout the brain are the same as in the rest of the body. Arteries, blood vessels, veins, and capillaries are all labels for the vital system that supplies the brain with nutrition and oxygen.

If a blood clot, or blood clots form and strokes result in any part of the path, neck or brain, oxygen will be cut off and neurons and neuro-transmitters will be damaged. This may result in plaques forming in the electrical path causing memory loss and possibly memory loss diseases such as Vascular Dementia.

Because of damage done to the neurons and the synapse, the person with dementia slowly and systematically loses memory, control, and eventually has behavior and physical decline.

Persons with dementia diseases cannot change what is happening or how they deal with life. Family caregivers need to start an intensive and careful plan to build long-term care plans for the loved one as soon as changes are noticed.

Keeping the loved one independent for as long as possible is the first priority. However, realism is pertinent in making sure that safety is insured.

Taking care of another family member takes organization, participation, and respect for all members. Every member should have a role, however small or large in the process of care.

Brain Activity Starts with the Senses

Some content was previously published as an article on June 5, 2012 at Examiner.com by Clarice Cook

We take information in through our senses, through our eyes, ears, nose, and feel through our skin. In the Cortex, we think about what we have seen, heard, smelled, or touched or what has touched us. The message goes to the inner brain to be sorted out as to the meaning of the senses and to put that information together with other sensations or memories of past experiences.

Once the mystery is solved, the information may be quickly discarded in those first three seconds, or depending on the importance of all the data, it may be coded and stored for future reference.

Perception is not predetermined.
How information is recalled depends upon the perception that goes on within the inner brain about the event or experience. What we take in through our senses is selective based on our interest.

It has been determined through research studies that 100-people witnessing the same tragedy while standing in the same area can give 100 different accounts of what actually happened. Some may have recalled some of the same information, but each had a different opinion according to how they viewed the event.

Researchers believe this is because no one is born with specific viewpoints. Intelligence, how we interpret smells, what we see, what we hear, or what we feel is not predetermined at birth.

People born in the years of the World Wars may have a different take on life, politics, and religion than someone who was born and experienced Viet Nam and the more prejudiced years. Indeed, people who went through the same period may have argument with each other about events or the effects of world events.

Perception may change with experience.
As time goes on, opinions and memories may change. Older people may experience confusion and the indexing of the senses cues may become scrambled. The smell of warm cinnamon cookies may bring back past memories, but the person that baked the cookies may be lost to them. Our identities change as we change, but our foundations after birth may stay the same. Who we are may not be who we were if we allow ourselves to grow. Many adult children state that their parents are set in their ways. This may be because at some time in life, what is seen, heard, felt, or smelled is no longer going past into the Hippocampus to be processed. The older person more easily recalls the long-term memories and they may be scrambled. Newer things may be rejected.

Strong likes and dislikes are established early, but can be built on if we allow it. Taste of foods, etc. is learned over time as we are exposed. At some point in life, people may reject a food, even if they once enjoyed it, because they do not like the sight or smell of it. As people get to the end of their journey in life, their perceptions of a food they had learned to love may change as the senses change.

Smell is closely related to emotions.
If a person has an unpleasant experience while sitting in a restaurant where fish is being served, they may become nauseous if they encounter that smell again. If a mother is harsh or cruel with a child about having eaten too many ginger bread cookies, that person may not be able to stand the smell of ginger again.

Touch is essential for quality of life.
Touch is extremely important in that people who are never touched have isolation and social problems. These people are lonely, even in a crowded room. Persons who have been abused find it hard to allow someone else to touch them.

Feel is important to send signals in the form of pain when there is injury or discomfort. Over time, the sense of feel deteriorates and caregivers should be vigilant about detecting and reporting cuts and sores, especially on someone who has a dementia disease.

Hearing is important in communicating.
There are many jokes among the elderly and with family about the mistakes made in communication when hearing is deteriorating. However, it is no joke to the elderly person who feels isolated and becomes anti-social because of communication problems. Hearing for most people, especially men, starts to deteriorate around the age of 50 years old.

Hearing well is essential, however, sometimes older people reject hearing aids because remembering to put them in, to clean them, and to keep up the batteries, etc. is an added chore. When caregivers offer to help, the older person may feel that more of their independence is being taken away.

If there is rejection for using the hearing aids, a family caregiver might talk with the hearing doctor to make sure that the devices are working and fitting properly. If that is not a problem, the care team might evaluate and plan how to encourage use of devices while preserving dignity.

Sight deteriorates faster than the other senses.
According to Cambridge Institute for Better Vision, 80 percent of what we determine to be true comes through the sense of sight. At 80 years old, we need 8 times more light to refract to the Occipital lobe in order to input the right information to the brain processes. It is important for the caregiver to make sure that lighting is good in the home to help prevent falls.

It cannot be stressed enough that medical health care professionals, caregivers, and families should be aware of how a person with dementia is acting in regards to sensed.

The brain needs to be challenged.
What the person sees and how it is processed with what is heard, smelled, or felt determines reaction. When there is damage in the neurons in the Occipital Lobe, the result may translate as something to fear, enjoy, and laugh at.

In yesterday's world with radio programs that only broadcast stories by voice, a person's brain was charged with imagining what the characters, place, and actions looked like. Now nothing is left to the imagination on T.V. and in movies. Therefore, the brain has no work to do. Less cells develop memories and more brain cells die for lack of activity.

Caregiver Steps
For a person who has memory loss and brain damage, encourage and present only television viewing that presents challenges to the brain, such as game shows. Comedy is good if enjoyed together. If watching positive discovery or travel shows, interact with them about the program. For most people who tend to become depressed easily or have anxiety issues it is best to discourage news, soaps, or movies that lull them to watch without response or interaction with others.

It is always better to play challenging board, card games, etc. However, lower expectations in the execution and outcome. Do not point out mistakes, criticize, correct, or argue. It does not matter if the game is not perfect. It does matter that the loved one, client or resident is using the senses and brain.

Use the games and educational videos and shows as tools to reach and stimulate those areas and lobes that are still viable.

Music is also a good way to reach those stored memories to dance (either in the chair or standing) for exercise and to stimulate the hearing. Use appropriate songs that are joyful and might bring memories of the time in which they were young. Use soothing music for times when agitation is high.

References
 The Brain and Five Senses Slide Share at slideshare.com
How the Brain Makes Sense of the Senses by Faith Bryne at psychologytoday.com and The Cambridge Institute for Better Vision

NOTES

Chapter Three -Overall Brain Function and Nerve System Interaction

Part of the Content from 'Cerebrum brain function and nervous system interaction as published February 2012' by Clarice Cook in Examiner.com

Although there is no guarantee that the most intelligent people will not get a memory loss disease, research shows that risk for Alzheimer's and other dementias can be reduced. Quality of life can be drastically improved with brain training.

According to the Alzheimer's Association at Alz.gov, learning every day is important to keep the brain functioning. In learning how the brain works, new brain cells are being used to reduce memory loss, and improve the storage and retrieval system.

The dementia brain may still be able to learn.
Remember that the part of the brain that has not yet been affected is still producing new neurons. Every opportunity to surround and present a group or one person with new and old activities can produce astronomical results, one cell at a time.

When doing an old activity, add a new component for learning. It may or may not seem to have an effect. However, when running that information back later, the person or persons may have an unexpected recall.

When a person is moved to a different hall, it may take some time to learn how to find a new space; however, the new path to walk in order to get to that room eventually becomes habit. If that area of the brain is damaged, help most likely will be needed each and every time.

It is extremely important that caregivers use patience, listen intently, and give a person with dementia plenty of time to process the new or old information. Use simple directives and never, ever tell that person that it is the second or third or more times the directions have been given to them.

In an activity, patiently show the group or one person how to do something by example. Then be clear, but understanding when guiding them through it. Never expect too much. Remember the process is important. The result does not matter. The praise should be for the effort and that person's interpretation.

The Central Nervous System
The central nervous system connects and runs throughout four upper lobes and inner and lower lobes. It is structured with neurons (nerve cells) and synapses (connectors). In the brain, neurotransmitters send information impulses along electrical pathways, processing and storing memory.

Even though the paths interact with all other areas in some way or another, some functions happen and communicate more with one lobe than with other lobes. In the Cerebrum (upper brain area) are the four major lobes.

Higher functions happen in the Frontal Lobe
Behind the forehead, higher functions control the intelligence by which the human makes choices, and sets forth actions for daily life.

On the left side of the brain of the Frontal Lobe, intellectual activities happen such as

-understanding and analyzing abstract thinking (such as Mathematics)
-reasoning and problem solving in daily life, -absorbing, collecting and using verbal skills,
-control of aggressive behavior,
-sexual behavior activity,
-decision making and voluntary movement.
-The right side of the brain is credited with creative activity. ---

Sensory awareness happens on the right side in activities such as
-visual perceptions,
-spatial orientation,
-musical abilities
-and other creative abilities

Studies have not proved left-handed or right-handed persons more intelligent or creative than the other. However, it has been determined that in most cases, all activity on the left-hand side of the body is controlled by the right side of the brain and most activity in the right-hand side of the body is controlled by the left side of the brain.

Sensory awareness is in the Parietal Lobes.
The Parietal Lobe area communicates a great deal with the right side of the brain to interact with sensory perceptions. It is located behind the Frontal Lobe. Taste, hearing, speech, sight, and feel are prevalent in this part of the brain. Perception of an experience through the senses in the Frontal Lobe affects the emotions occurring in the Temporal Lobe. The results are interpreted below the Cortex in the Hypothalamus.

In the Temporal Lobe area, emotions run high.
Part of the Temporal Lobe is involved in the limbic (inner base) area of the brain. Interpretation of language and awareness and discrimination of sound makes this lobe a major area of the brain. Emotions run high with such activities as

-feelings of love, that work with the right side of the Frontal Lobe

-anger and aggression that interacts with the left side of the Frontal Lobe

-compulsive behavior that works with the left side of the Frontal Lobe

-sexual emotions that interact with the left side of the brain for sexual behavior and with the Parietal Lobe for the sense of feeling

The Occipital Lobe is at the back of the brain in line with the optic tract
In review: The major functions in the back of the brain are to receive, interpret, and discriminate vision activity. Association with other lobes with information from the Occipital Lobe is important for memory processing and putting together information, such as, things seen with things heard and felt.

Perception in the brain of a person with dementia
For a person with dementia, perception as it is interpreted through what the brain processes, interprets, and remembers is the truth. If they do not perceive or remember it, it did not happen that way or it did not happen at all. If another person points out the reality, it can become a frustrating, humiliating, and argumentative confrontation.

Remember that if an event or request is not a harmful situation for the person with dementia or to others, then it does not matter. Let it go, change the subject, distract the person, and find laughter. Let it be their reality.

To learn more about the brain and memory processes, check out the video online at Medline Plus.com and Alz.org.

References
Mayfield Brain Clinic, National Institute of (not Mental) Health, Medline Plus - Brain and Nerves

Caregiver Quiz
Which is true based on the information in the above chapters?

-If a dementia patient becomes disinterested in activities they once enjoyed, such as reading, the family or primary caregiver should have the patient's eyes checked.

-If a person with dementia becomes irritable with interaction and conversation, the family or primary caregiver should have the dementia person's hearing checked.

-If a person misinterprets communication, it could be that connection to temporal lobe has been interrupted.

-A caregiver should preserve the dignity of the person with dementia by going with the flow, the change of conversation or agree with the perception of that person as long as it is safe for all concerned.

-All of the above.

NOTES

Chapter Four- The Cerebral Cortex – The Thinking Wrinkles

Some content is extracted from articles written and published by Clarice Cook at Examiner.com. This chapter is in review and further explained.

The Cortex is the wrinkled outer layer of the Cerebrum. This area is what has been called the 'Thinking Wrinkles'.

As it has been pointed out in previous chapters, each area of the Cortex takes care of certain functions. These functions happen in the approximately 100 billion nerve cells with connections that scientists call the "neuron forest." The brain cells, (the neurons or nerve cells), are where "tangles" occur causing dementia, such as, Alzheimer's disease.

The Cortex is divided into four lobes, which are the most involved part of the brain. These lobes are the Frontal (forehead area), Parietal (top center), Temporal (front on either side at and above ear level) and Occipital (back behind the eye).

The fast and furious action between all lobes brings about storage of memory from experience, interest or intentional study and research, exchange of ideas, impulses and thought with association, and two way automatic and intentional action between lobes.

The Intellectual Frontal Lobe
The neurons and transmitters in the forehead area (Frontal Lobe) of the cortex of the brain is the management and executive center. The outer area (lateral) of the Frontal Lobe organizes and plans actions and learns new skills and ways of performing tasks.

If a person has Frontal Lobe damage in this area, any familiar task can be overwhelming and learning new tasks is impossible.

Repeated Actions
Since the Frontal Lobe interacts with the Temporal Lobe, a person who has Alzheimer's or perhaps another form of damage in this area, will get stuck on the last remembered step and repeat actions for old task over and over. For instance, a person may be making a bed and get to the step to put the top sheet or blanket on. Forgetting how to continue, they will stop, take the bed apart, and start over again. Sometimes the person will

play the action out, but often frustration and loss of patience creates chaos.

Caregiver Steps
If a caregiver or loved one is standing by when a repeated action starts, it is best not to stop the person abruptly. If the person becomes agitated, move in gently. Being careful to preserve the dignity of the person, give them value by distracting them to a different task, hobby or game that they previously did well. Make them feel that you or someone else needs them somewhere else. Sometimes just talking calmly and appealing to their need for companionship may effectively bring the person back to a more balanced state.

If the person persists and becomes upset at your interference. "No, No, I have to finish this.", redirect them calmly by something like, "Oh, I see that you have the bottom sheet on your bed." This may be the place that the person keeps stopping and starting again. Continue by handing them the top sheet. "Here is the top sheet." Encourage movement toward that task. Try not to interfere too much in that task, but just gently keep the movement going. When that step is finished to that person's satisfaction, hand them the coverlet if they stop again or seem confused. Continue with them until the bed is made.

Lack of Motivation
The center section of the Frontal Lobe motivates and generally encourages need to perform activity. If the neurons and neuron-transmitters are damaged in this area of the lobe, the person may seem lazy and unwilling to participate in life.

Caregiver Steps
The main goal of the caregiver is to maintain the person's dignity in any case. To belittle, or try to motivate a person by making them ashamed with disapproval is counterproductive. Realize that a person with Frontal Lobe damage may have broken cells and connections in the brain that limits motivation to move. Also, realize that one day there can be connection, the next moment the interaction may not be happening.

Continue with patience to present happy times, words that motivate, pictures or activities that stimulate and do not be discouraged if it does not happen soon enough or not at all.

If the caregiver is a family member or family primary care person, talk with the health care professional about the possibility and/or type of damage in this area. If the caregiver is an agency or otherwise professional, come to an understanding with the family about how care can best be given and how to make that person with brain damage feel valued.

Inhibitive or Inappropriate Actions
The curvature part of the very front of the Frontal Lobe area is the Orbitobasal area. This is where behavior is controlled, monitored, and moderated for healthy people. It is the area where inhibitive action over programmed data takes place.

NOTES

Chapter Five -The Receiving Occipital Lobe

Eyes convert light into electrical impulses that are passed to two different lobes for interpretation. The sensory information is processed and divided into two different distinctions, visual acuity, and perception. Visual acuity is the job of the eyes and perception is interpreted by the Occipital and the Parietal Lobes (above the Occipital, behind the Frontal).

The Occipital Lobe decides the color, (in the left side) shape (right) and movement (right), and then the parietal lobe receives the information to determine perception of what is seen.

Caregiver Steps
Dementia persons with poor eyesight may need help in keeping eyeglasses clean and in wearing them. Since eyesight plays a big part in coordination, walking and perceiving what is seen, caregivers need to assist in helping with these tasks. Perception of what is seen is a big issue, especially for persons with Lewy Body Dementia. If the client or resident normally wears glasses, take notice and make sure glasses are clean and that the person is wearing them.

The Perceptive Parietal Lobe
Between the Frontal Lobe and the Occipital Lobe, the Parietal Lobe at the top back of the brain cortex puts gathered information into a 'perceived' file." There are dominant and non-dominant assignments in this lobe as well.

Tasks for putting letter or word data or calculations together in proper order happen in the dominant side of the Parietal Lobe. Movement skills are also perceived in this area and perception of personal space. Report any changes in sight to the responsible party.

Note: If a person has problems with tasks assigned to the Parietal Lobe, it is not necessarily an indication that there is damage. A case in point is Apraxia, a condition of impaired memory of movement. Dyslexia (left to right awareness) is also a condition that is not a diagnosis of damage to the brain.

On the non-dominant side of the Parietal Lobe, visual information is received from the Occipital Lobe and combines information into a 3-D perception of what has been seen. Damage to this lobe may suffer from a symptom known as visual agnosia. The affected person may not be able to recognize objects, faces or surroundings and interpretation of what is seen may cause episodes of hallucination.

For instance: If damage has occurred in the non-dominant Parietal Lobe, but not in the area of the brain for hearing interpretation, a person may not recognize a friend by sight, but if the friend speaks, recognition may be immediate.

Perception of external objects and space is processed in the non-dominant portion of the Parietal Lobe. People with damage in this area may not be able to calculate how far away a fork is to a plate, or may knock a cup over when trying to reach for it.

Caregiver Steps
It is imperative that caregivers make a note of any changes in motor or memory skills and relate these differences to health care providers or primary care family members. However, when dealing with one on one situations, three keys for a caregiver is understanding, patience, and respect.

Listening and alertness with patience is number one with communication and interaction with a person with any cognitive impairment.

For instance, if a person is becoming frustrated when trying to speak, say, "It's o.k. to take your time." If the frustration continues, change the subject quietly and with respectful words.

It is up to the caregiver to decipher communication through circumstance, situation, body language, and to know the basic needs of the client or loved one. The caregiver can sometimes say, "Oh, I think I understand", and recite to the client or loved one a short sentence that gives understanding. Many times, the person will be delighted that you were able to bring about a resolution.

-Do not let enough time pass that will allow the person to become too frustrated, but be patient and let the person know that you are listening.

-Never make a person feel like there is "something wrong with them." There is indeed nothing wrong with whom that person is. Let them know in your interaction, in your demeanor, body language and in the way you communicate and present yourself that you value them as a person and that the impairment is human and not something they can control.

-Never overwhelm the client with too much information or words. Every approach, every interaction and every chore or goal should be simplified and personalized to that person's ability.

-If a person is hallucinating, at first agree then distract and bring them back to a real place. The episode may stop and then begin again later. Treat each episode as if it were new and repeat the agreement and then distraction. ("Oh, I understand, isn't that something?" or "Margaret will be coming inside shortly. Let's go to the living room so that we can answer the door bell.")

Caregiver Quiz–

-What are three keys for successful communication with a person suffering from dementia?

-What actions with patience is number one in interacting and communicating with someone with cognitive impairment?

-What methods can be used to decipher communication?

-How can a caregiver show value in a person with cognitive impairment?

-Name some ways that interruption of the senses can affect behavior in a client.

-What is the main consideration in dealing with an inappropriate situation caused by the person with cognitive impairment?

-How can the caregiver deal with an episode of hallucination?

Chapter Six -The Limbic System - The Gatekeeper to the Brain

We all are aware of the tiny computer chips and cells where it is possible to store billions of bits of information. Consider this and think about the fact that the entire brain is about three pounds in weight and the Limbic Lobe itself has areas the size of peas that store, integrate, and communicate enormous amounts of data and run all operations for the body and brain.

In other chapters, anger outburst issues and caregiver steps are discussed. Information will be addressed in this chapter to explain the location of how the temporal lobe interacts with the Thalamus, in particular, the Hypothalamus in controlling emotional actions and reactions.

The Limbic Lobe is located in the base of the brain area and sits over the spinal column. The structures of the Limbic System are part of the Thalamus, the Hypothalamus and each are closely aligned to the Frontal and Temporal Lobes.

The Hypothalamus is an important emotional center that controls hormones that give us emotions like happiness, unhappiness, and anger.

The Thalamus is a type of information clearing tract. The Thalamus tract leads from the Spinal Cord to the Cerebrum. An arching tract leads from the Hypothalamus and Thalamus to the Hippocampus.

The Indexing Hippocampus

The Hippocampus is a tiny hub that indexes (sorts and filters) memory data and sends the completed 'file' to the various and appropriate areas (file cabinets) of the Cerebral Cortex for long-term storage and possible recall.

For the person without brain damage, the process of listening with interest, associating the bits of data, and taking action helps the healthy brain to store events and new information through the hippocampus.

Recall Activities

In persons with short-term memory loss, such as is the case for persons with irreversible dementia, data cannot reach the Hippocampus to be processed. Therefore, even daily activities cannot be recalled the following day or within the next hour. Even though the long-term memory may still be in the storage areas, recall is impossible if the tracts in the limbic areas or the Hippocampus itself are damaged. If the storage areas are damaged, the information will be gone altogether.

Caregiver Steps

For many older people, pleasant recall of stories and past times bring a great deal of pleasure and enhance the quality of life. When first entering the home, meeting the family and reviewing the health care plan, take mental note of how the client views taking those verbal 'walks down memory lane.'

For veterans, it may be advisable to stay away from certain areas or questions about their war lives. However, if the conversation is voluntary, be a good and unbiased listener. If frustration escalates with the telling, try to distract without devaluing the storyteller.

People who have been victims of abuse or war tragedies in their country may or may not want to talk.

Looking at photos, scrapbooks or other historical items may have an older person telling and re-telling the same story. The caregiver or family member should remember that it is best to listen as though for the first time. If the story changes, do not point it out. It is their story, their reality and it does not matter about facts.

If a person seems disinterested or frustrated about telling stories, keep conversation to the present day with light, fun, easy conversation and with lots of laughter.

Example: A professional caregiver points out old pictures of family and friends to the client. The client is in a bad mood and says, "You don't know those people. I don't need to talk with you about them." The caregiver apologizes and says, "What would you like for lunch?"

Sometimes it is o.k. to become quiet and let the person breathe, turn on some appropriate music (not hip-hop or similar genre), and sing or talk about something funny. Again, it is important to know that person in order to choose interaction.

Above all, do not take any actions personally. It is the disease. The best way to turn negative situations around is with patience and levity.

Avoiding Frustration
To argue, tease or point out inaccuracies with any person with dementia, aging or brain damage is counterproductive and exacerbates the disease or condition.

The wise caregiver or loved one can avoid angry outburst by watching for cues to agitation, by distracting the person with something positive, by keeping experiences, conversation, and events simple and by encouraging laughter.

Remember that it is the disease, not the person. A person suffering from dementia has no control over his actions. It is the caregiver who can monitor and who can make the difference in the outcome. In most cases, any frustration is the result of something the caregiver did, sometimes without realizing it.

For instance: (Moving too fast, approaching from the back or side, etc.)

Approach slowly from the front.
Speak with respect, adult to adult.
Look at the person eye to eye.
Give the person space with respect to hearing ability.
Speak clearly and succinctly.
Use few and simple (not baby talk) words.
Never reprimand the adult, always suggest/redirect.
Never argue with an adult with dementia.

Stress and the Aggressive Amygdala
In the center on both sides of the hippocampus, the small egg shaped Amygdala is where perception of stress issues gather. Integrating the factors and communication from the Frontal and Temporal Lobes, the Amygdala creates feelings of anger through images that are tied to the feelings. The neuro-transmitter hormone, acetylcholine is thought to be most active in the area.

According to The Lancet, January 11, 2017, studies, a study of 293 patients made a connection between stress and an increased risk of heart disease and stroke. The various research studies targeted activity with "a combined PET/CT scan of the brain, bone marrow and spleen activity and inflammation of arteries." It was found that "the amygdala is more active in people with post-traumatic stress disorder (PTSD), anxiety and depression..."

A continued series of studies confirmed these findings and it was found that "those with higher amygdala activity had a greater risk of subsequent cardiovascular disease and developed problems sooner than those with lower activity."

The Lancet report also suggested that in negative stress situations, the amygdala signals a biological action on the arteries that causes development of plaques that become inflamed. It is known that plaque and inflammation of arteries is a danger for heart attack and stroke. It is also known that Vascular Dementia is a result of plague and inflammation of arteries in the brain.

According to a Lancet sub-study group with a small number of 13 with PTSD patients, a psychologist measured levels of C-reactive protein, an indicator of body inflammation. The persons with the highest levels of stress had the highest levels of amygdala activity with more signs of inflammation in blood and artery walls.

This report would indicate the danger of stress and the connection of stress in the Amygdala. In summary, plague and inflammation are caused by stress. It can be safely surmised that negative stress can lead to dementia in the brain.

In addition to the information from this report, we know that in the healthy brain, the chemicals responsible for stress levels are dopamine, serotonin, and norepinephrine. These are dominant in the limbic area where the Amygdala resides. These hormones are thought to balance the nervous system and create balance. Negative stress can lower these vital components and put the neurons in jeopardy.

Defusing Aggression
If aggression cannot be avoided or if the caregiver steps into an already escalated situation:

-Stay to the side of an ambulated person, and only approach them if necessary.
-Keep a safe distance, but block the way in cases where the person may be in danger by trying to escape to the outside.
-Suggest to homeowners or facilities to disguise doors to the outside with posters, banners, and wallpaper or paint colors.
-Avoid talking to the person or adding any element that can 'add fuel to the fire' and is unnecessary.
-Be empathetic; agree with them regardless of what they say.
-Speak with a calm and soothing manner, when
verbal communication is necessary.
-Allow the person to express needs without reproach or comment.

Deter the path of someone who is trying to go to dangerous areas or escape outside by standing beside them and moving sideways and into the space without touching them. Direct them in this way to turn into a corner and follow a wall back into and toward a safe area. Presenting safe pathways helps to bring them back. Then create an activity or create a scenario that makes that person want to stay where it is safe.

For instance, a person with Alzheimer's has reached a wandering stage. She is on a constant watch. In the home, the family has installed door alarms and has 24 hour in home caregivers. Keeping the client interested in activities is no longer an option, because the client is no longer interested in anything except leaving and going 'home'. Nothing is familiar anymore, even for the client that may have lived in that home their entire life.

The caregivers in this instance should use the above tactics of distraction, calm speech, and listening, in a way to ensure safety and serenity for the best quality of life. Go in conversation to the place in that person's mind. "Where do you live?" "Who lives there?" Then suggest that it sounds wonderful and that "We have reservations for tonight." If there is still a determination to leave, suggest getting up to go "pack for a fresh start in the morning." Then walk with them around the house pointing out old pictures of family and friends. Ask questions about the pictures and get them to talk about old times. In this way, the client can be re-oriented to the reality of being "home."

The Lancet report can be viewed at eurekalert.org.

NOTES

"Remember, Remember, Remember: What does it matter? If it is not important to the immediate safety or welfare of the client or the persons surrounding that client, change the direction, the conversation, or actions of the situation in a positive way. Deal with any event with productivity and safety first in mind. This path will lead to high quality of life and that is the ultimate goal." Clarice Cook, CDP

The Basal Ganglia

Around the Thalamus are clusters of nerve cells that initiate, manage, and integrate movement for physical balance, emotions, motivation, control of eating and sleeping, storage of emotional memory, and control of libido. In addition, this is the area where the sense of smell is processed.

Damage in the brain that breaks the tract to the Basal Ganglia or damage in the Basal Ganglia could result in tremors, and stiff, rigid body movements with a shuffling gait, such as is the case with Parkinson's disease, Lewy Body or Parkinson's with Lewy Body. Sometimes Parkinson's disease in the physical sense leads to dementia, thus Parkinson's Dementia is irreversible.

A person with Lewy Body disease may have illusions (images that are not there.) This may be due in part with the impaired vision they may have.

Caregiver Step- Delusions and Illusions

Go with the flow, agree with that person, and then distract them. Never tell a person that he or she is seeing things or they are wrong about what they are seeing. Remember: It is their reality and that is all that matters. If they see it, it is there. If they do not see it, it is not there.

If a person with any type of dementia has illusions, consider this: It is probably like trying to watch a 3 D movie without the 3 D glasses.

Caregiver Step- Physical Challenge

Caring for a person with Parkinson's with dementia requires physical care training in addition to understanding and training in dementia care. Certified Nursing Assistants, Certified Medical Assistants, Physical Therapist, and others with knowledge of how to assist someone with physical disabilities have a good foundation for success. Knowing how to work with persons with developmental disabilities is also helpful.

For any person who is considered a fall risk, it is imperative that caregivers work closely with the physical therapist care plan in helping the client with any exercises, with walking equipment and with ambulating through the home.

For some persons with irreversible and later stages of dementia, it may not be possible to train them on the use of new equipment. If health care professionals make this determination, more attentive care than normal may have to be taken to keep the client or family member safe.

It is important not to be overly protective, but aware and prepared. Being in partnership with a physical therapist is important for safety while protecting independence.

The Smell Sense in the Hippocampus
The 'olfactory' (smell) processing area is a close neighbor to the hippocampus and limbic area, leading scientists to believe that this is why smell has a large impact on emotions and memories.

If a memory can be recalled, it may be because there are still links in undamaged areas that are triggered by certain smell clues.

Hunger, the urge to eat, the desire for foods that were once favorites, can be affected by loss of the sense of smell. This may be one factor in why loss of appetite brings on the failure to survive and the rejection of nutrition, medication, and liquids.

Caregiver Steps
It is unlawful for a caregiver to force food, nutrition, or medication on the client regardless of their condition. Any treatment actions must come from the health care professionals (doctors, practicing nurses, etc.)

It is recommended that clients be offered pleasant surroundings, pretty place settings for meals, and good nutritional food to encourage eating activity. However, if the client refuses, the caregiver needs to log that as 'Refused' and not make an issue of it. Sometimes waiting a while and reintroducing the offer may lead to an acceptance. The same goes for medication. In home, professional caregivers are, by law, not allowed to dispense medication. However, the law does allow that the client be "reminded" that they need to take the meds. If the client refuses, the caregiver should log it as a refusal and make the medical health care professional aware that the client is not taking the medication. However, it may just be a matter of waiting awhile and then reintroducing the reminder. Make it the client's decision in a respectful way. Sometimes a "no" actually means "yes."

NOTES

Chapter Seven-Caregiving Techniques:
Understanding Brain Center Function and Interaction

Some contents from "Understanding Brain Center Function and Interaction published in Examiner.com, March 19, 2012 by Clarice Cook

Professional and family caregivers and higher functioning patients sometimes feel inadequate, even with communication training, in understanding what is going on in the brain of persons with memory loss. While the medical health care professionals are responsible for this knowledge and for treatment based on diagnosis, it might be helpful for others involved to learn a little about the facts behind the mystery. This chapter clarifies the pathways to a greater extent.

Neurons and Synapses
As discussed in other chapters, the neurons and synapses in the outer cortex of the cerebral_lobes interact with the center of the brain to pull pathways together, move the perception, logic, and recall clues to appropriate areas of the brain for storage or to deliver information for response.

The center of the brain communicates with the neural activity in the Cortex of the cerebral lobes. The lobes in the center of the brain are the Thalamus, the Sub-thalamus, and the Hypothalamus. These areas connect and make possible the activities in various lobes of the Cortex or "wrinkled thinking" outer area of the brain.

All incoming sensory pathways except for the sense of smell are processed in several groups of cells in the Thalamus. Motor skills (the ability to move or automatic responses), visual (sight) skills, auditory (hearing), and association (ability to assimilate) are communicated here between the cortex and the fibers that contribute to appropriate responses.

Sub-thalamus
Sub thalamic nuclei, located in the Thalamus are concerned with motor activity and have connections with the Basal Ganglia. (Basal Ganglia are four grey matter masses located deep in the cerebral hemispheres.) Hearing and sight functions are included in the processing through this area.

The hypothalamus consists of masses of neurons and associated tracks.
This area is where sleep activity, pituitary gland activity, body temperatures, emotional reactions and other responses are regulated from the frontal and temporal lobes. Headaches, thyroid problems, sleep disorders, eating disorders, and reproductive disorders may be the result of hormonal dysfunction.

Four of the brains most important balancing hormones, Serotonin, Dopamine, Norepinephrine, and Acetylcholine are responsible for many functions and are located in the hypothalamus. Functions such as blood pressure, emotional balance, thyroid, and adrenal activity are affected by the stability of the hormones.

The caregiver's role in assisting enhancement and interaction is important.
The most important things to remember for a caregiver in helping someone who has a brain injury or dementia disease is to maintain patience, understanding and use compassionate, but impersonal reactions.

Because damage to areas that deal and interact with emotions, logical thinking and appropriate social skills, a client may display anger, inappropriate sexual advances, and some may strike out in abusive ways against caregivers. Learn ways to back off, stand aside, and verbally diffuse these explosions. Just being quiet with slow, kind body language sometimes works.

The caregiver can research and find creative ways to help the client sleep at the very least through sleep cycles of one and one half hours or more.

It is best to find ways to enhance (not force) nutrition. Encourage physical and brain activities as planned by physical therapist and dementia or brain specialists.

References

NIH The Brain Understanding Neurobiology How Neurotransmitters Work
Brain Anatomy, Brain Tours psycheducation.org

Chapter Eight -Cerebellum and Brain Stem – Coordination of the Brain and Body

Understanding of what is happening in the Cerebellum means that the caregiver has knowledge of the affected person's basic motor and non-motor function or malfunction. Knowledge makes it possible for the caregiver to adjust and help the client to adjust by finding alternative ways to do things like move and speak.

The Coordinating Cerebellum

Located behind the Brain Stem, the Cerebellum allows us to perform activities such as dance, talk, run, and do other things that require coordination.

The Cerebellum consist of two hemispheres with a thinking area (Cerebella Cortex), center motor skill area (deep Cerebella), Nuclei and trunk and branch like white matter (arbor vitae), and branches (Cerebella Peduncles) which attaches to the Brain Stem.

Equilibrium in motor skills, such as, balance and muscle movement and non-motor skills, such as, speech, and cognitive skills such as, daily planning, speed in understanding information, memory and other cognitive skills receive interaction in the Cerebellum

Sense of personal space and judgment in movement, muscle control, and overall coordination in response to commands from the higher cortex are all involved here.

Speech Skills

Speech skills involve both motor and non-motor coordination. Multiple muscles of chest, mouth, throat, and tongue are involved with the very act of forming words. Recall is needed to find the right words and organize them in the proper sentence structure. Problem with annunciation of words (as in slurred speech) takes coordination of combination of letter sounds (phonics).

Caregiver Steps- Coordination and Motor Skills

A damaged Cerebellum or transmission of the information required for coordination in this area can cause obvious unbalanced actions and reactions. Outcome will depend upon the event of cure or permanent damage.

Caregivers play an important role in ensuring individually focused and compassionate understanding and help for persons and families who are living with physical and mental challenges.

Physical and/or occupational therapy is important in helping people who suffer from reversible damage to the motor areas of the brain stem and the cerebellum.

For instance: Strokes do not always lead to dementia or permanent memory loss. Some damage can most often be repaired with stringent occupational therapy. Depending upon the severity and the diligent work on the part of talented therapist and the patient, damage from strokes have been either reversed or compensated for after a few months to a year and beyond

Be prepared to follow professional's orders in the care plan for assisting a stroke victim with any walking aides. However, be aware that persons with limited cognitive skills may not be able to understand how to use a walker, cane, etc.

Some restraining aides require special orders and can be against the law to use. Even though a person has problems walking, it may be safer to hold hands with them or just be ready to assist when getting up and moving about the room. Just because it is inconvenient for the caregiver or others does not make it right to keep a person maintained in a chair or bed when the urge is there for them to move.

Caregivers need thorough training in how to hold and move down with a person to the floor in the case of apparent fall movements. In any case, follow instructions of the care plan set down by physical therapy professionals.

Co-ordinate with Therapists
Occupational therapists are concerned with the upper body and the function of the arm and hand movement to take care of daily task, eating independently, etc. Physical therapists work with getting the client to the

highest level possible in ambulating, (wheelchair, walker, independent ambulation). O.T. and P.T. require the client to exercise both in bed and throughout the home, etc.

Sometimes, in home caregivers may be asked to prompt clients in performing simple daily exercises according to a care plan, such as walking, lifting limbs, stretching or breathing, and relearning (when possible) activities of daily living. Those assigned to assist with these client activities should learn the correct techniques and ensure that the client is safe during the exercise.

Caregivers need to be able to assist and help those with irreversible damage to learn new ways to communicate or ambulate. However, in cases of dementia diseases such as Alzheimer's, deterioration will produce new changes every day. This requires that all persons involved in the care plan be one of acceptance and appreciation of each day, whatever it brings.

The Transmitting Brain Stem

The Brain Stem is composed of sections in the Midbrain and Hindbrain with Nuclei for Cranial Nerves. The Medulla in the Brain Stem controls respiration, heart rate, and vasomotor function.

The connectors (Interior Cerebella Peduncles) gather here from the upper portions of the brain and carry fibers to the Cerebellum from the Spinal Cord. Information from the upper brain also carries commands to and from the body to the brain.

Damage in the Brain Stem could render a person physically and/or mentally dependent short or long term. Alzheimer's and other memory loss diseases affect all organs, and muscles as well as motor skills.

Caregiver Steps
Before accepting positions with persons who have physical and/or mental issues and need help with the activities of daily living, plus certain health care assistance, the potential caregiver should take care to train and be familiar with the physical therapist plan.

Chapter Nine -Using Equipment Aids

Wheelchairs

Persons with physical disabilities sometimes need help with the use of manually operated or motorized wheelchairs. Learn how to make these safe in and out of the home.

-Make sure that wheel chairs are at an angle to a bed or chair before transferring the person. Ensure that the locks are set to avoid movement of the wheels during transport.

-Be well-trained one on one in how to safely pivot or otherwise transport a person with physical disabilities. Note that older people are prone to bruising, and bones and muscles are fragile. Be especially sure not to pull or tug on or under a limb on the weakest side of the body.

-Inspect the chair periodically for safety issues.

Canes and Walkers

Under all circumstances, avoid the use of throw rugs in a home where ambulation requires equipment or when motivating around the floors are difficult.

Follow any advice or procedure plans that are diagnosed by a physical therapist. Report any slipping of adjustments on canes or walkers.

For instance: Watch and walk to the weak side and behind the client when they are up and moving around. If a person starts to teeter, be ready to support. Have finger grasp under the gait belt to balance. If a person starts to fall, and it is unavoidable, help them down slowly by going down with them. (With your arms under the armpits and hands grasp in the front, break their fall and follow the movement down.)

First, make sure that a fallen client is secure. Then call for professionals to inspect that person for broken, cracked or dislocated bones or other damage. The professional may also determine the reason for the unstable movements that caused the fall.

It may be necessary and is recommended that an incident report be filled out and signed by all concerned. File with the appropriate professionals.

Gait Belts/Walker Belts
Special made belts are sometimes used for persons who are at risk for fall. Learn how to apply and use the belts to safely transfer or prevent falls. This training should be done one on one to understand safety fit and use.

Patient Transfer Boards and Sheets
Boards and special made sheets may be in use to transfer people unable to use their legs to get from chairs or beds. It is critical to learn how to set the boards up properly for safe use.

Taking Care of the Caregiver
Taking care of the needs of someone who has both motor and non-motor damage is a big undertaking. Caregivers should be in good physical and emotional shape with good training.

Caregivers should be as vigilant about their personal physical and emotional care as they are about the patient care. It takes someone with healthy physical and emotional strength to be an effective caregiver for persons with physical disabilities.

Caregiver Quiz

-What are the two brain areas that are responsible for motor skills?

- What are three pieces of equipment that a caregiver should know how to use with a physically impaired person?

-What are some steps in walking with a fall precaution client?

To learn all the steps to transferring clients and other safety issues, go to MedlinePlus.gov

Chapter Ten -Degenerative Brain Diseases - Processing and Storage

Contents from "Degenerative brain diseases processing and storage" published in Examiner.com, March 22, 2012 by Clarice Cook

Degenerative brain diseases can be from many causes, and can imitate many different diseases of the most powerful organ of the human body. Dementia, which is related to the decline of language, memory, visual, spatial and judgment skills in the person that everyone may have known differently, can change drastically.

The first sign of dementia most likely will start with short-term memory loss in an area that continues to escalate to include long-term memory.

Long-term retention starts in the Entorhinal Cortex and interacts to the center where the Hippocampus sets the data up for storage (long-term memory). If a connection is broken or the data is not coded correctly, the information never makes it to storage and most likely what is heard, seen, felt or perhaps what the person smells is lost.

Sorting and storage of memory happens in about three seconds at the most.

A normal brain will process the information in the adnominal cortex, between the two frontal lobes, and pass it on to the center 'gray matter' for storage in the Hippocampus in the Hypothalamus area. It is much the same as with a computer that processes the information through the ram and stores it on the hard drive.

The brain can hold seven things for processing at one time. In those three seconds, only that which is perceived as important to remember is chosen for storage.

Clogged arteries and/or neurons and neuro-transmitters prevent connections.

Sometimes, members of the family have a hard time understanding that the person with memory loss is not being inattentive or rude. In fact, the inner portions of the brain between the two temporal lobes that controls hearing, seeing, logic, and assimilating new information are deteriorating.

Damage is preventing appropriate sorting and bringing together information and understanding. If the input is not gathered properly, it will disappear from memory.

Normal aging happens differently than the process of the damaged brain.
With degenerative diseases, the brain loses its ability to repair damage in the processing area of the brain where new brain cells build new memories. For instance, the diseased Alzheimer's brain can no longer learn new skills and as the disease progresses to a stage three and four, the hippocampus is also involved and long-term memory becomes impossible.

Older persons with normal brains can still retrain by learning new things; however, older neurons can be lost faster than new ones can be developed. The learning process may be slower than it is with the younger brain, but the capacity is the same. New skills can still be processed in the endocrinal and stored in the hippocampus.

Early health care and detection is essential for longevity and quality of life.
Denial and/or apathy can prevent people from brain training, physical exercise, refraining from the use of tobacco and drug misuse, eating and drinking properly and finding natural relief for stress. Since memory loss and dementia symptoms can start as early as forty-five years old, scientist suggests that early attention to health care is a priority life style.

Fear that memory lapses could be degenerative can keep persons from scheduling and getting tested for memory loss diseases. Early detection can make the difference between fast progression and a better quality of life.

References
National Institute of Neurological Disorders and Stroke Ninds Cerebellar Degeneration Information

US San Diego School of Medicine Department of Neuro Sciences Neural Degenerative Disorders

Chapter Eleven- Expectations and Habits

It has been determined that all humans form habits from birth. Those habits stay in memory forever unless we systematically and intentionally write over them. It is the same with a computer file that we no longer want. We can delete the file, but it will stay there until a new file writes over it. In a person with dementia, recall of certain habits may be gone forever, but the person can form new habits over that space where the old habits once existed. Scientists have also learned that function in the brain lobes may not be transferable in people with memory loss.

If a part of the brain where sight information resides is injured, or in cases of impaired vision or blindness, the other senses may take over and be useful in satisfactory performance. This can be the case for persons with dementia if brain training is available without high expectations.

Family caregivers and sometimes professionals can be extremely hurt when the loved one or client reacts in hateful and aggressive ways. Caregivers should be ever mindful of sudden changes in personality or moment to moment demeanor.

Remember that the chemistry in the brain is being controlled by the disease. Curb expectations and remember that it doesn't matter as long as the loved one or client is safe.

I have heard caregivers say, "Oh, she knows what she's doing." My answer is. "Maybe. But one thing is definite, she no longer has control over her actions. Her logic is not your logic." Therefore, it is the duty of the caregiver to insure safety first to all concerned. Nothing else matters.

When a loved one or client is being nasty, remember that the person is hurting. That person cannot make logical sense of what is going on and it hurts too much to not be able to control actions or situations; therefore, that hurt may be mirrored onto someone else. It's always easier for anyone to not accept the responsibility for guilt over mistakes or inadequacies.

We all have to train ourselves to face our mistakes and accept responsibility for our choices. A person with dementia or other brain disorder may not be able to make choices any longer on a rational level. Therefore, they feel guilt for everything, right or wrong, but it's overwhelming to accept responsibility to change it.

Chapter Twelve -Effects of Dementia Diseases in the Brain and Family Understanding

Content from Effects of dementia diseases in the brain and family understanding was published in Examiner.com by Clarice Cook June 29, 2011.

The effects on quality of life and family understanding depend a great deal on understanding brain function. Understanding how Alzheimer's and other dementia diseases affect personalities and lifestyle is important in order to deal with the day-to-day changes.

Degenerative brain diseases are Alzheimer's , Pick's, Vascular, Huntington, Creutzfeldt-Jakob disease, Frontal-Temporal Lobe, and Parkinsonian type dementias, such as Lewy Body and others. Part of the difference is damage from protein in the originating and affected part of the brain where the information is processed. Another difference is the chemical component that is affecting the normal flow and processing of data.

The first sign of dementia most likely will start with short-term memory loss in an area that continues to escalate. In Alzheimer's, memory loss can be slowed down and sometimes stabilized in the early stages. Reversible dementias, such as brain tumors, strokes, depression, dehydration, surgery, metabolic disorders, side effects, infections, nutritional deficiencies circulatory disorders, substance abuse, head trauma, toxic factors, and others, can sometimes be halted and methods used to heal the damage. However, as with all diseases, early detection is important and follow-up treatments are crucial. Not all damage can be repaired, however, in most cases; the effects can be halted and slowed down. While everyone forgets from time to time, people with an irreversible brain disease will begin to have functional difficulties that gradually take away abilities to deal with life.

Often people with dementia protect their independence and consider others intruders and enemies that suggest that they need help in any way. Denial is persistent and trust becomes a problem for them.

Processing information in the Entorhinal Cortex

According to Wikipedia.org
Definition of *entorhinal*

> : of, relating to, or being the part of the cerebral cortex in the medial temporal lobe that serves as the main cortical input to the hippocampus

Explanation according to the Merriam Webster dictionary: **entorhinal cortex (EC)** (ento = interior, rhino = nose, entorhinal = interior to the rhinal sulcus) is an area of the brain located in the medial temporal lobe and functioning as a hub in a widespread network for memory and navigation. The EC is the main interface between the hippocampus and neocortex. The EC-hippocampus system plays an important role in declarative (autobiographical/episodic/semantic) memories and in particular spatial memories including memory formation, memory consolidation, and memory optimization in sleep. The EC is also responsible for the pre-processing (familiarity) of the input signals in the reflex nictitating membrane response of classical trace conditioning, the association of impulses from the eye and the ear occurs in the entorhinal cortex

Sometimes, members of the family have a hard time understanding that the person with memory loss is not being inattentive or rude. In fact, the inner portions of the brain between the two temporal lobes that controls hearing, seeing, logic, and assimilating new information are deteriorating. Damage in the entorhinal cortex is preventing appropriate sorting and bringing together of information and understanding. If the input is not gathered properly, it will disappear from memory.

Stored memory in the Hippo-campus

A normal brain will receive information from the senses sent to the various lobes and assimilate in the entorhinal cortex, between the two frontal lobes, and pass it on through for storage to the original section of the brain by the hippocampus. It is much the same as with a computer that processes the information through the ram, (random memory), and takes it to a processing program that sorts it and then stores it on the hard drive when the operator gives the save command. All components must be working correctly to ensure correct processing and storage.

Short-term memory loss and long-term retention

Lost retention is especially frustrating for the spouse of a person with dementia. There is often conflict when the afflicted spouse remembers the past vividly, but cannot remember a trip to the movies the night before. Persons with early onset dementia can recite tiny details of a childhood vacation, but may not be able to remember to lock the door when leaving the house or to take medications on time.

Normal aging versus the damaged brain

Normally, as we age the brain loses its ability to repair damage in the processing area of the brain where new brain cells build new memories. As it is with all cells in the aging or diseased body, neurons are lost faster than new ones are replaced.

Older persons with normal brains or with reversible dementia may be able to retrain the brain by learning new ways of doing things. The learning process may be slower than it is with the younger or normal brain, but new skills can be processed in the entorhinal and sent to the hippocampus to store.

Alzheimer's and other irreversible brain patients can no longer learn new skills. As the Alzheimer's disease progresses to a stage 3 and 4, the hippocampus and gradually the back of the brain in the parietal are also involved and all memory becomes impossible. Research and education about dementia diseases can lead to early detection and treatment for a better quality of life and better family relationships.

Chapter Thirteen -President Reagan: Facts about Diagnosing Alzheimer's and Dementia Diseases

Content of "President Reagan: Facts about Diagnosing Alzheimer's and Dementia Diseases" was originally published February 19, 2011 at Examiner.com by Clarice Cook

Ron Reagan, Jr. wrote a book depicting his perception of his father, President Ronald Reagan and the link to Alzheimer's. According to the book, Ron believes that the President had Alzheimer's in the first term of office.

According to Alz.org, in the Reagan presidency years, a firm diagnosis of Alzheimer's required an autopsy of the brain with an electron microscope and testing of proteins after death. At that time, the only evidence while alive would have been based on symptoms and not a true diagnosis.

Health care professionals for the President may have had access to information that would have indicated the onset of dementia. However, many forms of dementia share some of the same symptoms, such as Dementia with Parkinson's, Pick's disease, Fronto-Temporal Dementia, among many others. (Note: Parkinson's disease is not a dementia. However, person's with Parkinson's can develop dementia, thus, Parkinson's Dementia.)

Alzheimer's research has since brought about technology and knowledge that proves that persons with early stages of the disease can be very intelligent in different ways. Dementia symptoms can affect language, visual or spatial abilities or judgment in addition to memory and physical skills. However, forgetfulness or a temporary lack of judgment, loss of concentration or focus is not always a sign of dementia.

Although the Alzheimer's Association educates the public on symptoms that may be related to memory loss, the actual diagnoses for any dementia disease should be assigned to trained health care professionals, who take all the necessary tests to make a firm determination.

Alzheimer's brain deterioration is not inclusive or predictable for every person

Persons with dementia diseases do not exhibit the same symptoms, stages or the same level of intelligence. Having early-stage Alzheimer's does not mean that a person is incompetent, unstable or are unable to make life decisions. People with early and later stages of all types of dementia have been known to live alone and conduct business with minimal assistance for many years. However, it i s important that the daily living be monitored closely for important changes and that decisions be made for increased in home assistance or for a move to an assisted living facility. Families should have a long-term care plan set up according to need.

Brain exercises, medication, and training have been shown to slow down progression and improve Alzheimer's quality of life.

Some persons with memory loss deterioration called Mild Cognitive Impairment or amnesic MCI, may be more capable of conducting business and making life decisions than someone without the disease and may die of physical causes before dying of Alzheimer's. Not everyone with Mild Cognitive Impairment will go on to develop Alzheimer's. Others may quickly need assistance and seem to perish in a few years. This can depend on when the diagnosis was made, the condition of the person, treatment, and other factors unique to that person.

Dementia Practitioners can conduct cognitive skills, memory test, and physicals.

Complex tests can be performed by dementia experts to give health care professionals the precursors for determination of further examination. Cognitive skills test determine ability to function on a daily basis, memory test determine degree of short term or long-term loss, and physicals determine if motor skills or organ functions have been affected.

Technology can determine dementia diagnosis accurately

Experts run imaging techniques, such as, angiography, CAT scans, and MRIs on the brain of a person who has been exhibiting symptoms such as confusion, behavioral changes, hallucinations, or memory disturbances. The scan of a brain suspected of Alzheimer's will show white, empty spaces and other abnormalities compared to a normal functioning brain.

According to the National Institutes of health in an article at Alzheimer's Disease Education and Referral Center, Alzheimer's Disease Genetics Fact Sheet, Early Onset Alzhiemer's testing in persons with a family history could determine inherited traits for the disease. In these tests, people as early as in their 30's who have the genetic mutations, have a 50/50 chance of developing Alzheimer's in their life time.

Read more at www.nia.nih.gov/alzheimers/publication/alzheimers-disease-genetics-fact-sheet

If genetic predisposition diagnosis and treatment for people such as Ron and Michael Reagan and others determined the certainty of development of Alzheimer 's, they might be able to start treatment sooner. However, many people might want to leave it to chance and not know. As of this date in 2017, the treatment programs have already been used in other countries, but recent reports state that the FDA has not approved it. It could even be possible that scientist will discover a vaccine, for possible causes such as viruses. Science has started to move quickly in new discoveries. What may be relevant today may be old news tomorrow.

All persons with dementia should be treated with dignity and respect and without prejudice or judgment.

Join the discussion about Alzheimer's diagnosis and learn more about Alzheimer's, or to support research for Alzheimer's or volunteer to join the fight against dementia diseases. Check out ALZ.ORG

Resources and References

Surgeon General.org Mental Health: A Report of the Surgeon General Alzheimer's Disease

National Institutes of Health NIH

Major Milestones in Alzheimer's at Alz.org

Alzheimer's Association, Mild Cognitive Impairment

Help Guide.org Alzheimer's Disease Signs , Symptoms and Stages of Alzheimer's Disease

Mayo Clinic Early Onset Alzheimer's

Alzheimer's Association. What is Alzheimer's

NOTES

Chapter Fourteen -Type of Dementia: Does it Matter?

Some content was published at Examiner.com on June 15, 2012 entitled 'Dementia type diagnosis Memory loss symptom health care differences' by Clarice Cook.

Researchers have found that there are similarities and differences in all dementias that may require the same or different therapies or medication treatments. Testing and case studies have shown that the development of different symptoms, the genetic makeup and other medical conditions and history may require different treatment at different times.

Symptoms happen differently or at different times for each type of dementia. Symptoms for one type may be different or overlap. Sometimes people have more than one type of dementia. Caregivers should know what is possible or probable in the present and future in order to be able to recognize behaviors and to communicate, interact and plan for the best possible quality care for the loved one or client.

Many symptoms are the same or similar while others are exclusive of the type of disease. This is because of cause and nature of the deterioration of the brain cells and path.

Evaluation should be ongoing.

A few minutes to an hour or so in examination and oral testing can provide a false positive diagnosis. This is because patients may be stressed and confused by being among strangers and in a strange place. Therefore, at every stage, the health care team may order blood test and other more clinical procedures to check for the type of protein, hormones, or other causes that may be responsible for that particular type of dementia. Health care professionals should also monitor the person in their familiar environment with family, friends, and caregivers.

It matters that the professionals have the correct information in order to help determine the type of dementia. Patients, family and paid caregivers need to provide the health care team with details on symptoms, reactions to medications, all present and past health issues, and family and personal health history.

By providing the history, the physicians and dementia practitioners can use this knowledge to determine genetic possibilities or other causes for dementias such as Alzheimer's, Lewy Body disease, Vascular Dementia, Dementia with Parkinson's, or Frontotemporal Dementia.

Alzheimer's Versus Lewy Bodies
Persons with Alzheimer's disease go through three stages of the disease over a possible period of twenty years. Symptoms can start as early as the early forties.

Symptoms for Alzheimer's Dementia include a progressive loss of recent memory problems of language, abstract thinking, and judgment that are unusual for that person. There is also the presence of depression or anxiety, personality and behavioral changes and disorientation and confusion to time and place. Lewy bodies dementia starts out with some similar and some different symptoms and become more pronounced as time goes by. Some people start with memory or cognitive disorder that may resemble Alzheimer's disease, but over time two or more symptoms distinguished as Lewy bodies may appear.

The symptoms that are different from Alzheimer's include the on again, off again occurrence and levels of cognitive skills, attention and focus, alertness and changes and decline of motor skills. In Lewy bodies, there may be visual hallucinations, sleep apnea or sleep disorder called REM.

Both diseases may create all night walking, wandering, hoarding, and a determination to go "home."

Lewy Body dementia symptoms have some different clues.
Persons with LBD or Lewy Body dementia may display patterns that may seem like they are sleepwalking or acting out dreams while awake. Although the actions seem to be hallucinating, the person may have a severe sensitivity to medications for hallucinations. Although some persons with other types of dementia may also have these indicators, Lewy Body has a significant chance for this symptom.

Over time persons afflicted with Lewy bodies throughout the brain will suffer from cognitive, physical, sleep and behavioral features, however, some features of this type of dementia are exclusive.

A small group may actually show substantiated signs of hallucinations as a part of neuropsychiatric symptoms. There may also be behavioral issues and unusual problem solving episodes with complex mental activities. This combination of symptoms is a leading diagnosis of Lewy Body dementia.

In some cases, the sleep disorder can precede the dementia and other symptoms of LBD for many years. Other sufferers may start out with a motor skills disorder leading to diagnosis of Parkinson's and later develop dementia and other symptoms common to LBD.

Parkinson's Versus Lewy Bodies
Parkinson's disease does not always lead to dementia. Lewy Body is a dementia, but does not always accompany Parkinson's. However, tremors and out of control motor skills are a symptom of both Parkinson's with dementia and Lewy bodies, sometimes leading to misdiagnosis.

For many family members, the difference between Lewy Bodies dementia and other dementia diseases, such as Alzheimer's is not important. All that matters is that the loved one is suffering, the relationship is being altered daily, and for whatever reason, the goal is to make that family member happy. However, quality of life may be improved with the right medication for a correct diagnosis.

Some symptoms of Lewy Body and Alzheimer's are overlapping. Some symptoms of each disease require different treatment for the best success for quality of life. The most exact diagnosis requires extensive MRI's and other x-rays that go beyond the verbal testing by doctors. Neurologist should be consulted and family caregivers should be vigilant in finding out what the test results reveal and insist that the proper treatment be administered.

Alzheimer's symptoms show up in many dementia diseases.
According to the Alzheimer's Association, the earliest sign of Alzheimer's disease is short-term memory loss that goes beyond normal temporary lapses of recall.

Other changes might include:

-inability to plan and function (banking, dealing with shopping, cooking, dressing or appointments)

-taking longer to perform tasks that were normally routine

-time and place confusion

-trouble with judging distance in driving

-difficulty with reading or understanding directions

-writing, repeating speech, misuse of words

-inability to retrace steps in finding lost items

-poor judgment in dealing with business dealing and money exchange

-suspicious, depressed, anxious, and fearful and withdraw from social activities.

A brain scan will show tangles of the neuro transmitters caused by plagues of the tau protein and progressive brain shrinkage.

Lewy Bodies symptoms are similar in many ways.
Lewy Body Dementia is the second fastest growing memory loss disease diagnosis. As stated in the previous text, LBD has some very similar and some very distinct differences.

Memory loss is not typically the first symptom of persons diagnosed with Lewy Bodies. Lewy Bodies can be diagnosed as dementia with Lewy Body or with Lewy Body and Parkinson's disease. Sometimes Parkinson's symptoms come on at a later stage. Sometimes Parkinson's is the first diagnosis.

While persons with Alzheimer's decline and stay in stages of symptoms steadily for long periods, declining to the next stage, Lewy Body symptoms are progressive as well, however, incidents fluctuate from minute to minute and day to day. While Alzheimer's patients may test poorly in the mental cognitive test in beginning stages, persons with Lewy Bodies are apt to test in the normal range.

Symptoms that start differently from Alzheimer's may include fluctuating:

-attention deficit

-ability to execute familiar tasks

-alertness

-hallucinations that are real and in detail

-spontaneous events similar to Parkinson's

-difficulty in recognizing family and friends

Persons may have increased incidents of falls and fainting, spatial disorientation, dysfunctional depth perception, unexplained loss of consciousness, visual disturbances, object disorientation, and hallucinations. A shuffling gait when walking, loss of motor skills, incontinence, and drooling may also be apparent.

A correct diagnosis is important in order to set up successful treatment for good quality of life.
In addition to technology in diagnosis, professionals may look at different combinations of symptoms that are specific to Lewy Body.

A correct diagnosis is difficult in hourly visits in unfamiliar surroundings and with strange people. It is important for family members and those close to the patient to relate to professionals all symptoms and concerns in activities of daily living, instances of depression, aggression, and changes in cognition and other concerns in order to arrive at a correct diagnosis.

Top four known dementias: Vascular, Alzheimer's, Lewy Body, and Fronto-Temporal
Vascular Dementia is caused by series of mini or major strokes that cut off oxygen and nutrition from the brain. This causes damage to the arteries and veins that feed the neurons and neurotransmitters. The neurons and

neurotransmitters collapse if the arteries and veins cannot be repaired. Not everyone who had strokes develop dementia and sometimes the brain can reconnect in the damaged sections. Vascular Dementia is diagnosed after it is determined that the damage is irreversible. Symptoms of Vascular Dementia are similar to Alzheimer's.

Alzheimer's is a neurological disorder caused by a necessary but over phosphylated tau protein that hardens the memory tracks and storage cells. The track knots and breaks, preventing memory from traveling to the synapses, which may also be damaged, and then progressing throughout the brain. The disease can start early and continue for as long as twenty years.

Lewy bodies are abnormal proteins that deposit throughout the brain causing deterioration of brain function by destroying dopamine and acetylcholine. Loss of these important message-distributing chemicals important to efficient brain function results in both unique and similar symptoms to other types of dementia. Illusions are frequent due to the interruption of sight perception.

Fronto-temporal dementia is most common for personality and inappropriate or compulsive behaviors that are not normal for that person. A person with affliction in the frontal and temporal lobes of the cortex most often experience euphoria and or apathy. As with many dementia types there is a decline in personal hygiene and lack of awareness. There are several forms of Fronto-temporal dementia involving communication problems and motor skill damage.

Mixed Dementia

In recent studies, researchers have found that more than one type of dementia can be present in the brain. A person with

- beta amyloid formation of tau protein from Alzheimer's,
- Lewy body attacks on vital memory carrying chemicals,
- obstruction of oxygen and nutrition through veins and arteries in Vascular disease
- and/or destruction of motor skill chemical of dopamine in Parkinson's with dementia may be all or part inclusive in a person with dementia.

There are many other dementias and more are being identified every day. Aging is not necessarily a certainty for "senility"; however, it is an added risk.

Education for Planning and Development of Care

By educating family members and caregivers, and professional health care providers, persons with dementia can get better quality of life. Planning is essential for financial and care issues. Home security can be insured if modifications can be made to coincide with the changes in capabilities of the person with the diagnosis.

Making the home safe is a progression as the person goes from self-care to assisted or total care. If families can anticipate the symptoms and have some sense of future decline, decisions can be made about the safety of the loved one in the home or whether to move them to assisted living or total care environments. Knowledge can alleviate the stress and frustration for the patient and for the caregivers.

There is a test to measure memory that can be a prerequisite for presenting for possible testing. This self-test is called SAGE and can be downloaded from the Internet

www.alzheimersreadingroom.com/2010/04/test-your-memory-for-alzheimers.html.

Caregiver Quiz

-What is the value of education on the symptoms of different dementias and what can be expected from each?
-Can there be more than one dementia present in a brain?

-What are the four leading irreversible dementias and what are their unique symptoms?

Chapter Fifteen-Preserving Dignity for Memory Loss Client or Loved One

Content from "Preserving dignity in care giving for persons with Alzheimer's disease' August 24, 2010 at Examiner.com by Clarice Cook

Preserving dignity is always a first priority with any client or loved one. However, when a person has memory loss and there is never to be any recall, such as in Alzheimer's disease, making that person feel equality and value is even more important.

Having said that: intervention that may work for one person may not work for another person and that same interaction may work one instance and not another. Changes are happening constantly. Moods, confusion, and acceptance are always on the move.

In the progressed stages, it might be perceived as trying to wake up from a dream, but never making it to full awareness.

Empathy is number one. Patience is an absolute necessity. Positive manipulation is forgivable; however, speaking adult to adult is always preferable.
An in-home caregiver shared a story about a woman who felt that she needed little or no assistance. At the beginning of the first shift, the caregiver asked the client to share what she expected her to do.

The client, Elouise stopped and thought for a moment. Then she said in an angry tone of voice, "I do have a lot to share. I can tell you that. But if I have to teach you how to do things, then you should be paying me."

Reaction to a client who is guarding her dignity, even though her family and doctors insist she have help, is like walking a tight robe. Maintaining composure, not making it laughable, but showing respect is crucial.

Showing understanding and empathy has a calming effect.
The caregiver calmly said, "Well, you've got a point. However, if you can think of me as a helping friend who is here to fill in until you feel like doing certain things for yourself, I would appreciate that."

Persons with dementia have an increased sense of fighting for control. Remember that if a person with dementia feels that family and friends are aware of the forgetfulness and do not trust them to be in charge of their lives, resistance prevents acceptance. It is important to give a person with memory loss a feeling of power over life situations.

Every person is different and every event and day varies, so the caregiver has to be patient.
This approach helped Elouise feel comfortable and in charge of her life and her home. As time went on, dementia became obvious and she became impatient with the fact that there were still people in her home doing the chores and making decisions.

More caregivers and hours had to be added. This can be particularly confusing for dementia clients. More people involved and going and coming into the client's space means more to remember. Persons with memory loss are overwhelmed with too many questions or information.

Setting up a large calendar with schedules written in black marker in a prominent place in the house is helpful for those in earlier phases of the disease.

Caregivers need to use positive manipulation.
As the brain atrophied, Elouise started to lose trust and thought people were taking her things. She started hiding items throughout the house during hours when there was no one there. The toilet paper was stored under the bed, and the toaster was found under a pile of blankets in her bedroom closet.

Once Elouise stored the items, the recall was gone for good, but she would become agitated if people were searching for things. Caregivers had to be extremely careful in looking for lost items.

The approach to offer help in finding them helped Elouise keep control. Caregivers used communication such as, "Oh this happens to me all the time. Sometimes it helps if someone helps me. Can I go along with you to help you look?"

Sometimes if the location of household items were known to the caregiver, one article was slipped into an obvious place when Elouise was in another room. In this way, she was delighted in finding the item herself.

Again, it is important to remember that every human is different and these same approaches may not work for every client or in every instance. However, with patience, attention to body language, extreme listening, and versatility, a caregiver can make the day in the life of a person with dementia a little less stressful and happier.

To learn more about care giving techniques for memory loss persons, check with ADEAR, Alzheimer's Dementia, Education and Referral Center at Alz.Org

National Institute on Aging-Caregiver Guide   NIH.gov

NOTES

Chapter Sixteen-Communication Tips: Alzheimer's and Other Dementia

Contents of Caregiver communication tips: Alzheimer's and other dementia diseases were published February 10, 2010 at Examiner.com by Clarice Cook.

According to the Alzheimer's Association of America, Alzheimer's Foundation at Alz.org,

-Alzheimer's is one of the most common causes of dementia.

-People with dementia do not necessarily have Alzheimer's

-Alzheimer's is not a normal symptom of aging.

Alzheimer's typically begins with short-term memory loss that lasts beyond the normal forgotten thought. In a normal situation, a person might rarely lose a line or topic in speech or the location of keys, etc.

There are common factors in onset dementia and/or Alzheimer's, in that recent memory loss is frequent. As the disease progresses for the Alzheimer's patient, long and short term memories fade away forever.

Symptoms in each person with a memory loss disease may progress differently from the onset.

-Never treat the client as a child. Remember to respect people with impaired brain function as another adult. In keeping sentences short and simple, it is not necessary to speak to another adult as a child. Do not use a singsong voice or call them "darling," "honey," or "sweetheart." Use their names.

-Annunciate clearly, but do not speak louder than is necessary for someone who may be hearing impaired. Knowing the person and the unique capabilities will be the guide for how to communicate with that person.

-Be respectful when monitoring medical intake. Watch to see that there are no odd-looking pills or pills out of order, but take care to be discreet in reporting or redirecting the client.

-Allow the person to be independent with activities, but monitor and discreetly report any safety issues.

Professional caregivers need to be alert to changes.

-Stay up to date and record changes

-Be prepared to adjust to client's changing needs.

-Keep in close contact with care plan log and/or family or Client Care Coordinator to be aware of gradual changes.

-Research ways to cope with mood swings, changes in personality, increasing bouts of suspicion, withdrawal from communication, and lack of interest in beloved activities.

Find ways to alleviate stress over memory loss.

-Clients may need constant reminders of medication times, appointments, and events.
-Report when client shows frustration with financial or mental task (ex: checkbook)
-Reassure client there will be help for forgotten task.
-Do fun mental exercises approved by care plan.
-Gently assist client to remember words and complete sentences.
-Encourage verbalization about frustrations, anger, or sadness.
-Empathize with client about feelings.

Communication with the client may become gradually more difficult.
On every visit, realize dementia clients may be confused with who and why there is someone else in the home.

-When entering the home or room, always make client aware early who you are.
-Check and avoid loud distractions and noises.
-Use a pleasant, not overly loud demeanor.

-Watch non-verbal body language (gestures, touch, and tone of voice)
-Smile and/or appropriately (but slowly) touch an arm or take a hand.
-Stay in front of client.
-Make eye contact.
-Keep a pleasant voice, but loud enough for hearing impaired.
-Speak slowly, clearly and annunciate words.
-Never argue with a client.
-Keep questions and words simple and clear to client.
-If the client gets frustrated, have them talk out feelings.
-Stay with one subject at a time.
-Be patient and wait for answers.
-Keep sentences simple and emphasize key words.
-Give directions one-step at a time.
-Focus on past memories, childhood, and encourage positive conversations about family times and legacy.

Respect the client or loved one as an adult.
Emphasizing respect, remember that although a person with dementia is losing learned skills to the point of when they were children, they are not children. Do not talk to a client with childlike verbiage and voice tonation. Treat them with adult dignity. If they do not understand what you are saying, be patient and calmly repeat in a different way what you said with annunciated, but not exaggerated words.

Caregiver Quiz

-What is the most important thing to remember in offering and administering care for someone?
- Name three ways to communicate with a client who is upset, angry, or confused?
-How do you communicate to a person who does not understand you?

Chapter Seventeen -Dementia Diseases: Brain Training Stabilizes, Slows or Prevents Memory Loss

Content taken from the article: Dementia diseases: Brain training stabilizes, slows or prevents memory loss by Clarice Cook and published in the Grand Rapids Examiner.com

Mental exercises are essential to keeping the brain healthy and to ward off dementia. Repetitive information helps with retention of already learned information. Brain exercises should be designed to learn new information.

Forgetfulness comes with age and is not always related to dementia. In normal aging, new brain cells continue to develop and it is up to the senior to use those neurons to learn. Learning new information can prevent, slow down, or stabilize dementia development.

The entire learning process consists of focusing on new information, seeking understanding, and depending on how it is compiled; the entire package will be stored for later retention. For the older person, this can be a slower process, but it is not impossible.

Active brain training should be a daily activity.
Learning new information depends on health and interest in the activity at any age. Brain training should be practiced on a continual basis. Protecting the brain starts early on in life. Older people have to be more vigilant about sleep, nutrition, exercise and other health care habits in order to have good brain health.

Visual exercising calls for logical brain cell connection.
An attempt should be made to retrieve any new information later. An example would be in reading an article of particular interest and focusing on a passage, a new discovery or new place to travel. In order to create recall, the brain must understand and analyze what is read, assimilate and then store it. Later in the next day or so, try to recall the information and confirm it by returning to the article and reading it again.

According to Dr. William Rodman Shankle in Preventing Alzheimer's, other exercises that require perception, understanding, analyzing, retrieval, and execution of information might be puzzles, word and number challenges, and brain games.

Writing is beneficial if it includes outside-in learning and processing new information. Creative writers can include research of areas, places and time and perception to make the story real. Articles require research to validate information.

People who watch T.V. to relax are not exercising the brain for new information. Examples of actively watching content for learning would be a documentary, travel or other educational channel such as cooking or home and garden network. News, political and financial reporting encourages discussion, analytic and further recall exercise. However, it is best to encourage positive programming to avoid negative stress.

Early evening after game time might be a good time for relaxing video's, a romantic or lighthearted movie, or a comedy such as "I Love Lucy."

Physical interactive games can be played in many ways.

Outdoor games such as golfing, baseball, basketball, and tennis are healthier overall exercises for brain training for older persons who are able to be physically active. In cases of persons with limited mobility, the new interactive sport video games offer participation from wheelchairs or standing and using the brain, arms, and hands.

For the evening, a good relaxing, deep breathing and yoga type range of motion exercise done to soothing music might help sleep.

Table card games and dominoes with friends and family enhance social interaction while training the brain. A variety of games installed on computers can be played with hand held devices. Internet brain games are available at web sites such as Alzheimer's Association Maintain your Brain Game.

Go to Alz.org, to train your brain with the brain game apps.

Chapter Eighteen -Alleviating Effects from Negative News

Content is from 'Caretaker's mental health tips: Adverse reactions to negative world news, published May 8, 2011 at Examiner.com by Clarice Cook.

Natural disasters, political strife, war, terrorism, children killing each other in schools or at home, foreclosures, and spouses murdering and abusing families are in the news every day. Seniors and disabled persons watch and absorb the traumas making personal conditions worse.

People with dementia do not have the logic or at the least are limited in the ability to filter out the reality of negative information. For example: If someone is killed in a car accident, Nellie may be certain that the person killed is her daughter because her daughter drives a white car just like the one on T.V. In reality, Sadie, her daughter lives 1300 miles away. Nellie's logical centers are damaged, and cannot bring her that reality.

Caregivers are faced with helping clients alleviate reactions to negative news reports.

Professional caregivers have a responsibility to forget personal matters and intercede with stressed out dependent persons. This may be extremely difficult and sometimes the caregiver may have to face and deal effectively with unfounded, adverse remarks and accusations. At times, the troubled client may gossip about the caregiver.

Recommended Reading: At Examiner.com, an article, "Caregiver tips - Understanding Aggressive Behaviors and Preventing Escalation

"No one can make you feel inferior without your consent." Eleanor Roosevelt

Caregivers must take a deep breath and deal with the situation in a polite and tactful manner. Taking the actions of a troubled person inside serves no purpose. Remember that the action by the client may be the result of causes, such as, stress over uncontrollable negative situations, medication, the disease, or low self-esteem.

Choose words carefully, address problems with kindness, and give the client control over his or her actions.

For instance, a caregiver overheard a client with low self-esteem complaining about the caregiver's work over the phone to a friend. At first, the caregiver felt the natural pain of hurt, because she was confident that her work was exactly as it should be. When the client got off the phone, the caregiver said in a kind but confident voice, "This is your home and you need to address me when you are dissatisfied and let me know what it is that you want me to do. Telling your friend doesn't help." The rest of the day went well, however, in some cases, it may have been better if the caregiver had said nothing at all. The number one priority is to preserve client dignity.

In this case, the caregiver was being defensive and calling attention to the inability of the client to interact in a socially acceptable manner. The client could have in turn become defensive and could have become irate. Instead, she started refusing phone calls and stopped communicating. When she was asked why she did not want to interact, she could not remember the incident, but she remembered the feeling. "I'm not good at it."

Especially with Alzheimer's patients, memory of what the person just did may be gone. If a person has been diagnosed or show symptoms of this kind of memory loss and does not remember their actions, it is best for the caregiver to forget it.

Care giving is more than about physical health.

Mental health plays a foundation role in the well-being of every organ in the body. Nerves connect to the organs from the brain. If a person is under stress, the whole body feels the effects.

Waking up in the morning with a heavy, pressured feeling in the chest, burning and aching in different parts of the body and an overall feeling of impending doom is described by many persons, both old and young.

"Forget the times of your distress, but never forget what they taught you." Herbert Gasser.

Reactions to troubling times seem to be the most phenomenal when they happen, but for the elderly, the future is short and the present uneventful. The past is dominant. Looking back through time, a senior who lived through many war times and can tell many stories of survival may still suffer depression and worry about what is going to happen for the children and grandchildren.

References

Health team Michigan State University. Patients caregivers' issues

Building Self Esteem -A Self Help Guide samhasa.gov pdf

Deakin.edu publications pdf -The Impact of caring on caregiver's mental health: a review of the literature Sally Savage and Susan Bailey

Caregiver Quiz

-After reading the above chapter, what would you do if you overheard a client bashing your work to a friend?

-What types of activities would you suggest for a person who loves talking about the past?

-How should you react to a client who disagrees with you or offers some obviously incorrect information?

-What are three activities that Dr. Shankle suggests for better exercise for logic and to relieve stress?

Chapter Nineteen-Verbal and Social Interactive Dementia Caregiving

Contents for 'Verbal and social interactive dementia caregiving tips' by Clarice Cook was published at the Grand Rapids Examiner website on June 28 2011.

After a care plan has been established by a highly-trained neurologist, determining capabilities is the next step after diagnosis in order to establish a treatment plan. Symptoms of memory loss occur depending upon which section(s) of the brain are involved or what chemical may be deficient. In early stages, only one area may be damaged. In some cases, interrelated sections or lobes may be damaged.

The caregiver must understand that the person with dementia is not being obstinate or frustrated out of choice. The brain dysfunction is ruling actions and reactions.

Verbal interaction for persons with dementia
Become familiar with the person's level of understanding, independence, and stage of dementia for better communication.

Because the Frontal Lobe behind the brain or other interactive lobes may be damaged, a person with dementia may be un-cooperative, rude or even combative.

-Caregivers should not take any words, actions or reactions personally.

-When a demented person makes a negative statement of frustration or hopelessness, the caregiver should reply with a paraphrase positively to affirm that the person's feelings are being heard.

-Don't give answers as advice or lecture the person in any way. Give short suggestions that might help and remember that the person may reject all alternatives. However, later the person may take the advice, if it is remembered.

-Speak slowly, simply, calmly and succinctly and refrain from using too many words.

-Speak directly to the person. Make eye contact when possible.

-When other people are in the room, involve the dementia person in the conversation.

It is best not to tell the person what to do, but to suggest or ask. Questions should be structured, depending on the level of understanding.

Example: For later stages of dementia. "Susan, it's time for a bath."

For mild cognitive impairment (MCI), and those with understanding and desire for independence, it may be better to ask questions. "Thomas, would you feel refreshed if you had your bath now?"

"Mary, I'm here to assist you with your bath."

"How do you feel about your bath today?"

Give them choices (but not too many) as to whether they want to have a bed bath, sit on a stool for a sponge bath, have a shower or tub bath.

Of course, all options depend on the person's capabilities and mood for the day. It is also a good idea to establish with the MCI person a day or so before first event of care, such as bathing, the best time of day and the preference of type of bath, etc.

For those more impaired, do not be surprised if the person says "no." This may be to establish independence or it could be that the responsible brain area is thinking in the reverse. "No," may mean "Yes." Continue to prepare the bath water and reword the question. "Your bath water is ready."

Personal activities of daily living should be done in a safe and unhurried manner. Time for people with dementia is slow paced and hurry frustrates them.

Social interactions for persons with dementia
Remember that most persons with dementia diseases need space and are confused by too much chatter and noise. Too many people in the home can be frustrating and cause confusion. Sudden actions, fast movements

or taking care of the person in a fast pace can set off anxiety and adverse reactions.

Outings should be limited to quiet parks or other peaceful places where the person can feel relaxed and comfortable. This may mean that family gatherings should be avoided if there are too many children or if there are boisterous activities.

If a person displays the need for activities, there are agencies and facilities that offer entertainment and interaction in organized programs with dementia skilled facilitators and activity teams.

For instance: Planting and watering flowers, appropriate music therapy, fun exercise and games standing or geared for persons sitting or in wheelchairs. The ideas are endless. No game has to be perfect to the rules. Persons in later stages may still be able to identify cards or suits. Some might be able to move checkers around a board. The act of doing is important for muscle movement or bringing out thought processes that are still present in the brain.

References

Everyday Life with Alzheimer's Alz.org

National Institutes of Health National Institute on Aging Caregiver Guide at Alz.org

Chapter Twenty- Modern Adversity Techniques

The original content of 'Modern adversity techniques to prevent caregiver burnout and preserve client mental health dignity' was published September 29, 2010 at Examiner.com by Clarice Cook

Dealing with difficult people can add to caregiver burnout. People who are sick, aging, suffering from a dementia disease or disability can be especially harsh due to no fault of their personality or control.

Chemical imbalances, medication, pain, confusion, and illness processes can come between the caregiver and the client or family member.

The number one no, no in negotiation is taking what the other person is saying as personal, regardless of the relationship.

-Detach the self from the anger and the frustration of the other person.

-Listen and try to understand the meaning and/or pay attention to the body language.

-Make eye contact and try to send a message of understanding and willingness to comply with their expectations.

-Agree and accept an alternative to what was expected, but work back around toward a point as close to center as possible.

A breakdown in negotiation will happen if one or both parties are too rigid to compromise. In the case of a cared for client or family member, for the sake of mental health, it is the responsibility of the caregiver to step back and realize that whatever the confrontation, let it go.

People can only control themselves (or not, in the case of dementia) and some things are trivial. The important goal is the safety and well-being of the client or family member. Allowing situations to become toxic is not safe for any member of the family or the professional caregiver.

Training for professional caregivers should include intervention techniques, such as those taught by the National Council of Certified

Dementia Practitioners (NCCDP) and Dee Mayfield, CDP, TIPs of the Mayfield Health Care Seminars.

Modern caregivers realize that the old methods of "reality orientation" do not compute in the brain of someone with memory loss or dementia diseases. The time is now and the past is nothing and trying to make the person face truth about the passing away of loved ones or retirement serves to create frustration and confusion.

Techniques of dismissal of problems and fears verbalized by a person suffering with confusion, disorientation, and anxiety have been updated in training. The NCCDP teaches professional caregivers how to give healthy assurance and validation to the aging patient.

Stress for the caregiver and the client or family member can be alleviated just by learning how to deal with adversity and agitation issues in difficult times.

Reference
National Council of Certified Dementia Practitioners

NOTES

Chapter Twenty-One-Understanding Aggressive Behaviors and Preventing Escalation

Contents of this chapter were published as 'Caregiver tips: Understanding aggressive behaviors and preventing escalation' at Grand Rapids Examiner.com by Clarice Cook March 15, 2011

Professional in-home caregivers face many challenges in dealing with aggression. In the home, care may require a great deal of counseling skills for which training is not always available.

In listening to the client, caregivers are not licensed counselors, but are there to listen, and show empathy without condescending or judging.

Professional caregivers should be trained to deal with aggression.
Sometimes an in-home caregiver may step into a situation of pending aggression, or in to the middle of a full-fledged incident. Even the most experienced counselor sometimes needs to call for backup. In the case of the professional in-home caregiver, a strong 24-hour agency on-call support system should be available to support caregivers.

Stay to one side and at a safe distance in front of an agitated individual, be relaxed calm and rational and maintain self-control. Move and speak confidently, but slowly. Do not let the person grab an arm or hand. If this happens, put a hand on top of the grip and talk firmly but with a controlled kind voice and language and work the hand out of the clinch. Distract and maintain composure. Do not make fast movements. Do not approach from the back. Remember safety first. Do not argue or disagree with a person with dementia or brain disorder. Talk the situation down. In an in-home situation, at first opportunity, get in touch with the in-home agency.

Detecting agitation and preventing escalation of aggression.
Detecting when there is a risk for aggression may help to head off a serious incident. If the client is feeling anxious and agitated, speaking about impending fear, or dread of real or imagined loss, the caregiver can take steps to ease the client's mind.

A client can become frustrated and upset about unmet goals or imagined fear. Depending upon the client's triggers to cooling down, the caregiver can head off escalation of anxiety. Staying calm and listening to the concerns validates the upset person and brings the client comfort in knowing that feelings are important. This approach creates trust. Allowing the client to talk it out in a calm and rational way helps them to solve the problems without incident.

-Notice if the client seems fearful or upset. Ask open-ended questions about feelings in a kind and caring manner. This means trying to get more than a yes or no from the person without badgering.

Great care must be taken to demonstrate genuine attention with the goal of bringing cheer to the person who may feel trapped and at the mercy of people who have stepped into guarded and personal space.

For some people, sudden movements or other approaches may trigger a defensive mechanism causing fear and an urgent need to defend. When attending patients or in home clients, the caregiver should let the client know beforehand each step of ambulation, assistance and bathing. Bathing is especially frightening and sudden water applications, such as in the shower, without warning can cause fear and panic that can escalate into an uncontrollable fight or flight reaction.

Report manipulative or intimidating behavior
Dishonest manipulation and intimidation can go either way. A client may be showing signs of dishonestly manipulating the caregiver or may convey feelings that someone else is manipulating them. The caregiver must be mindful of the situation and report any accusations or suspect dishonest manipulation as soon as possible.

Intimidated clients can show signs of fear, helplessness, depression or inability to function normally. Report any new signs of unusual behavior in the care plan. A professional can sort out whether the client is being affected by intimidation.

How to get help for the client
If the client tries to intimidate, manipulate or show signs of aggression, the professional caregiver needs to immediately report to the in-home care agency. It will be up to the agency to report behavior to the

family or health care team, who may work with geriatric or mental health care professionals for crisis intervention and counseling.

Online Resources and References

(Your Community) Mental Health and Substance Abuse Services

NIH Pub Med Assaultive behavior in giving baths

UCLA Semel Institute - Prevention and Management of Assaultive Behavior Review

Caregiver Quiz

-As a caregiver, what would you do if a client or loved one became extremely angry or agitated over a trivial or imagined incident?

-What are some defensive mechanism triggers to agitation, mistrust, and anger?

-What are the major roles for a caregiver in the home of someone with dementia?

-What is the real issue in dealing with an agitated client or loved one?

Chapter Twenty Two -Distracting an Angry Client with a Mission

When a dependent person is on a rampage, being aggressive, uncooperative, mean- spirited or otherwise difficult, a caregiver should look beyond the actions and find ways to defuse, deflect and distract. Never argue. It's useless to try to reason where there is no ability to use logic. A person that has interruption in the frontal lobe of the brain between the left and right brain will perceive the events of life much differently than everyone else. Inaccurate perceptions can create stressful reactions.

When a person with dementia is displaying aggression, it may not be from anger, but from a defensive reaction because of the following:

- confusion of what is happening to them in their disease,
- fear of persons they can't remember or never knew
- anguish of not being able to control themselves or their body functions,
- terror from the feeling of free falling in their world,
- anxiety of the overall loss of ability to connect with those around them.
- frustration of not finding words, not hearing, understanding, feeling out of the loop in a conversation
- embarrassment of having someone else helping them in their most private functions
- depression over loss of ability to make own decisions
- grieving of "death" of self and who they once were
- sad memory of family members or others who have died and the past becomes current

Use the three D's to develop harmony. Defuse by calmly listening, speaking only for safety or leaving the person in a quiet place to wind down. Deflect by changing or removing objects or self that seem to be the triggers for the actions. Distract by calmly bringing the person back to a safe place, singing, joking or just hugging and confirming.

The above tactics may not work every time and the caregiver has to be ready to change directions and activities to make things better and bring that person back to a calm safe place. Displaying happiness may not be appropriate for someone who is embarrassed or hugging should not be used when a person is in an aggressive state. Take time, go to a calm approach and work it out as a friend and partner in the process. Let that person feel accepted and loved unconditionally.

Treating each scenario appropriately can set the stage for how the rest of the day is going to develop. A person may not remember the event, the people in the event with them, or when it happened, however, the feeling may linger for a long time. A caregiver can effectively make that person feel safe, validated and happy in order to encourage a safe and happy environment. Sometimes the health care provider may need to prescribe an appropriate medication plan to control anxiety, and depression.

Find out more about how to deal with behavior issues in a person with memory loss. Check out the manual, "Memory Path Care Solutions- The Dynamic Caregiver", by Clarice Cook, available online at Amazon and Barnes and Noble.

This is a true story about fight or flight. The names and location have been changed to protect client privacy.

Harvey had always been a reserved even-tempered and intelligent man, always in control of himself in business and personal life. In his later stages of Alzheimer's, his dream world took the reins and his family had to set up a safety plan with in home caregivers.

One caregiver had not yet seen a fully-fledged and high out of control incident from Harvey. One day, Harvey got up from a nap and went to the bathroom. As he exited the bathroom door, he headed for the outside door without recognizing her. His eyes were glazed over and it was apparent that he was still in a sleep mode.

The caregiver shifted into distract mode and walked to the side and tried to move Harvey to turn around, all the while gently and calmly saying things like, "Lunch is ready and I'd like you to join me."

Harvey's brain was telling him to continue and this person was invading his space and interrupting that mission. He turned on the caregiver, yelling at her that he had to go to work. She said calmly, "Oh, you don't have your keys and you need lunch." By this time, Harvey had the door open and stepped out to his garage. The caregiver stayed close and quickly reached around and locked the door to the outside when Harvey approached it.

The very act of locking the door seemed to break the memory path in Harvey's brain. He stopped and started to de-escalate.

The caregiver stepped slowly and turning, she said, "Hello Harvey, it's so good to see you again. Would you lead me into the house and show me the kitchen? I hear that lunch is ready."

Harvey blinked, smiled, and walked ahead of the caregiver back into the house and to the table. The caregiver set breakfast up for him, all the while cheerfully attending his needs. Then she said, "I'll be right here if you need me." She left him and stood at the counter to chart the incident.

After a long period of sitting and thinking alone, Harvey turned and greeted the caregiver. "Would you have lunch with me?" The caregiver said, "I will." She sat with him, reading him simple jokes, and getting him to laugh.

Then Harvey started talking. The caregiver had no idea what Harvey was talking about most of the time, but it was apparent that he was living in his dream of working, making deals and solving problems.

She looked at him directly straight in the eyes, kept a pleasant persona and interacted with "Oh, I see." "I understand what you're saying." "How is your sandwich?"

Intermittently, Harvey would stop long enough to eat a bite. After a full hour and a half, Harvey stopped and said, "Oh, I bet I'm boring you with all my talk. I need to stop and let you get on with your work."

The caregiver smiled and said, "I love to hear you talk. You can talk all you want to. But if you're finished with lunch, I'll let you have some quiet time to yourself."

Harvey said, "Yes, you can leave now."

Of course, the caregiver did not leave. She said, "O.K. When I'm finished cleaning your house, I'll go." That seemed to satisfy him and he went back to his favorite chair to sit, doze, nap, and listen to his favorite music.

The rest of the day went beautifully. Harvey just needed to unload. The combination of broken memory pathways, and hormonal imbalance aggravated by the fact that he was refusing his medications was all contributing to his loss of logic and control.

In interacting with a person with dementia, family and professional caregivers sometimes are left with feelings of guilt after dealing with an incident. They go over the events and think about how they might have handled it better.

As she thought about the incident, the caregiver realized that Harvey might have been trying to communicate that he was concerned that doors were not locked. Harvey's caregiver thought, "Maybe if I had told him that his office was in the house and locked the door to the garage when I came in he wouldn't have stepped into the garage." It was also possible that all Harvey wanted to do was to step out into the fresh air for a moment. Whatever the reason, caregivers need not go into a second-guessing mode. The main goal is safety. Just remember that persons with dementia know the feelings and urgency of their actions, but no longer have the reasoning for their need for fight or flight or the logic to react correctly.

In truth, we as dementia caregivers need to realize our humanism and remember the safety rules to survival of fight and flight. Speak in short, calm, respectful, and controlled sentences. Distract them with other options.

Stay to the side and turn with respected movement helping them to change their space without touching them.
Assess their intentions without questioning them. "Can I help you with something?" is acceptable.
Follow and distract. Again, do not touch the client. Walk in directions around them that will encourage the person on a mission to change directions, if possible.
Encourage by distracting to break the mission of escape

For some clients who are at risk for fall, walk to the back and side in a position that you could steady or lower them to the floor safely in an emergency. This is the rule for any person who has a fall precaution. For a person with memory loss, the brain signals may be aggravated by a caregiver who is too close or trying to break their path of flight.

-Give them just enough space to be safe. Work in parallel with their direction. Put yourself in view of a door or lane of escape.

Many times, the client will come at you for an attack. The brain is directing them to remove the obstruction. Be ready to seek help if necessary. Most of the time, these episodes will only last for a short time, but in severe cases, they could last for a longer period.

-Stay out of the way of physical contact and out of personal space.

-Stay calm, keep talking and distracting with safe options.

In facilities, pay close attention to policies of getting help, if necessary. In the home, it is good to have contact numbers, a phone close by and emergency numbers on speed dial.

Always remember. It is a disease that you are dealing with, not the client or loved one as he or she once was. People with stages of memory loss have no control over the process that is occurring in the brain.

Caregivers can alleviate, distract, and avoid, but it is impossible to train or change the actions that are the result of diseases like Alzheimer's. The person with brain alteration caused by disease cannot come into reality. The caregiver must try to step into and understand the hazy and foggy world of dementia.

Also, remember that the above scenario might play out the same again or maybe not at all. Interactions to distract might work with one person and not another. The caregiver must be ready to use whatever safe, respectful, and understanding approach necessary to keep the client from harm or distress.

Caregiver Quiz – Managing anger, frustration anxiety or attacks in persons with cognitive impairment.

-Name three ways to alleviate persons with an episode of anxiety.

-What are three ways to de-escalate an impending anger episode?

-What are the four ways to keep persons safe in a fight or flight situation?

NOTES

Chapter Twenty-Three - Risk Factors for Dementia from Other Disease or Medical Conditions

Contents of 'Exploring the risk factors for dementia from other disease or medical conditions' were published at Examiner.com by Clarice Cook on June 19, 2011.

While it is true that not all dementia is a diagnosis for Alzheimer's, symptoms that are a result of diseases and medical conditions may eventually lead to AD. Since Alzheimer's is irreversible, it may be prudent to get expert testing by two or more experts to see if memory loss can be diverted or if symptoms can be treated.

Inadequate nutrition, lax exercise, smoking, and other harmful lifestyle choices that lead to blood flow and oxygen starving diseases, such as stroke begin in early years. Stroke is a contributor to dementia.

Detecting memory loss risk factors

William Rodman Shankle, M.S. M.D. and Daniel G. Amen, M.D. are authors of Preventing Alzheimer's. Shankle and Amen state that preventing Alzheimer's will help "understand and reduce your risk factors, learn how to detect problems early, obtain an accurate, prompt diagnosis, and choose the most effective treatment."

According to Shankle and Amen, degenerative diseases contribute to damage to neurons that can never be repaired. Over a period of time when about one third of the number of neurons decline, memory loss that does not return will begin a series of dementia symptoms that can develop further into Alzheimer's.

Many things can be done to prevent the ending results of dementia and Alzheimer's. Diet, exercise, and the very act of learning about new things are some of the habits that lead to better overall health.

Vascular Dementia (VD) Syndrome and Subcortical Vascular Dementia (SVD)

According to Dr. Ralph Sacco in Dementia/Alzheimer's Weekly, Young America on the Road to Dementia, life style habits start at an early age.

In chapter one of Preventing Alzheimer's, Dr's Shankle and Amen submit that "hypertension, diabetes, heart disease, stroke, tobacco smoking, excessive alcohol and a sedentary lifestyle" can all contribute to Vascular Dementia Syndrome, which can develop as early as 50 years old. 15 to 20 percent of dementia cases can be attributed to VD.

Sub cortical Vascular Dementia affects small blood vessels in the brain areas below the cortex. This progressive dementia normally starts after age 50. Diagnosis for this disease is hard to pinpoint because memory loss is not consistent. Sometimes the person can remember facts even when the event occurs under stress. At other times, recall is gone. If there is a drastic change in someone who formerly had good memory and recall, it may be suspect of small, undetected strokes.

Prevention and maintenance of new brain cells
Research studies show that up until the age of 75, new brain cells can be used to create new memories in persons in early dementia stages. After age 75, repeat activities can be retained and memory loss delayed with exercises, nutrition, alleviation of stress and a happy lifestyle.

Everyone has occasional memory lapses when under a lot of pressure causing stress or because of sleep deprivation. This could be the result of new cells dying because of not being used, disease, and drug or lifestyle abuse. Total loss of recall, change in personality, loss of desire for normal activities and other concerns indicate immediate need to be tested for dementia.

Resources.

Medicinenet.com WebMD live transcripts Stopping Alzheimer's Before It Starts

A book - Preventing Alzheimer's by William Rodman Shankle, M.S., M.D. and Daniel G. Amen, M.D. ISBN 0-399-15155-9 Putnam

Chapter Twenty-Four -Stroke and Dementia

Not all persons who have strokes have irreversible memory loss; however, stroke can be the cause of Vascular Dementia.

Serene Branson: Migraine Aura and Stroke Symptoms

This chapter was originally published at Examiner.com on February 19, 2011 by Clarice Cook.

It was reported on February 18, 2011 on CBS, the Early Show that Serene Branson's gibberish episode on Sunday, February 13, 2011 was not the result of a stroke as many speculated. Speculators through U-Tube and other Internet media quickly diagnosed that Serene had a stroke. However, there are other causes that can bring about headaches, visual impairment, changes in behavior, numbness in the body, disturbances in speech and other symptoms normally attached to stroke activity.

A top-rated health care team did extensive blood work and brain scans and determined that Serene's episode was the result of Migraine Aura, causing a short in the brain thought to speech.

Migraines are headaches that signal brain dysfunction.
The definition of migraine is from a French word derived from two Greek words meaning half and skull. Some dysfunctions may affect parts of the cortex, but other sufferers may have abnormalities occur in the layers surrounding the skull.

The classic migraine sufferer may have attacks that usually start before age of 30 and occurrences often decrease with aging. Sixty per cent of sufferers are women.

There may be ignored warnings days or hours before onset that can include mood and behavior changes, inability to sleep, change in appetite and doctors might diagnose a fluid imbalance if consulted.

Migraine Aura is one headache form of brain dysfunction.
Migraine Aura is described as a sensation shown in brain scans as a light or glow that starts at the base and surrounds the brain. According to

Headaches.org, migraines with aura are a "manifestation of neurological symptoms."

In rare cases, slurred speech, headache, weakness and overall "not feeling well" symptoms are diagnosed by health care professionals as Migraine Aura. Stress, overwork, loss of sleep might be causes that lead to the disturbances, such as what Serene Branson experienced.

According to Michael Bjorn Russell and Jess Olesin, it is possible to have Migraine Aura without the headache that Serene Branson described with her session of temporary speech impediment, numbness, and other symptoms.

Migraine Aura, although rare, runs in families. Daughters most likely will experience episodes in younger adult years, if mothers have the gene,

According to Christian Lampl and S. Marecek, from the Department of Neurology Psychiatry, Center Linz General Hospital, Linz, Australia, migraines can be a risk and precursor to the event of strokes. Further, studies show that the risks of strokes in persons with migraine with aura are greater than without aura.

Brain dysfunction associated with migraines has some symptoms of stroke
An episode of temporary speech impediment caused by migraine activity can resemble a stroke. Patients may have unilateral pain, nausea or vomiting, bowel problems, tingling, numbness, and other complaints associated with strokes. Complaints are varied, depending on the location of the dysfunction.

Strokes are the first layman thought when Migraine Aura symptoms occur.
Strokes most often occur in people over 65. The description of a stroke is an acute blood supply disturbance of the brain. Incidents of stroke can range from subtle and obscure to dramatic and obvious to the untrained eye.

Symptoms, such as, slurred speech, headache, and weak limbs can also be testimonial to other conditions. Test need to be performed by specialist to diagnose an actual stroke. Speech impediments from stroke are usually permanent or last for long periods.

It is possible for people to return to a functional degree and a better quality of life. If medical attention, care and therapies are applied, and if the patient is determined and vigilant, amazing stories of strength and function has been reported from some post stroke victims.

For the sake of caregivers, family members and for self, it is important to seek medical attention as soon as symptoms start. Continuing to try to function normally when severe headaches or other symptoms occur could be fatal if stroke or a bad result from a brain dysfunction such as Migraine Aura should occur.

Online Resources and References

Strokes: Cerebral oxygen extraction, oxygen consumption, and regional cerebral blood flow during the aura phase of migraine L Friberg, J Olesin, NA Lassen, TS Olsen and A Karle, Department of Clinical Physiology, Bispebjerg Hospital, Copenhagen, Denmark

Stroke.ahajournals.org

Migraine and Strokes: Why do we talk about it? Christian Lampl, S Marecek Dept. of Neurology and Psychiatry Pain and Headache Center General Hospital Linz Australia Migraine.org

Headaches.org The Complete Guide to Health Headache Types

Department of Neurology, Glostrup University, Glostrup Denmark, A Nesographic Brain PDF. Oxford Journal Michael Bjorn Russell and Jes Olesin

Chapter Twenty-Five- Gabrielle Giffords and Caregiver Understanding of Brain Injury Symptoms

Contents from Gabrielle Giffords: "Caregiver understanding of brain injury symptoms" published at Examiner.com August 4, 2011 by Clarice Cook.

While a continuing dementia may or may not become an issue for a person with brain damage, symptoms may sometimes be similar. Persons with brain damage are considered to have a possible irreversible dementia, at least to some degree.

Interaction with someone with brain injury or atrophy sometimes takes extra patience and focus. Having some sense of what is going on within the person's brain may help a caregiver to understand better how to assist the client without causing more frustration than is necessary.

Symptoms of brain damage or atrophy vary according to area affected and the interaction between the different lobes.

The left side of the brain rules the right-side motor skills, and the right side operates functions on the left side. A caregiver should be ready to assist the person to balance the right side for left side brain injury and left side balance for a right-side brain injury.

Frontal Lobe motor skills and speech
Abstracting from the University of Arizona report of Gabrielle Giffords, who was shot by a mad gunman in January, 2011, the right-side deficits of a sense of balance and motor skills indicate that damage on the left Frontal Lobe side of the brain, in the forehead area, could contribute to her right side weakness and speech problems. Her amazing patience, resilience and cordial attitude proves that her personality or emotional and interactive skills were not changed in the trauma.

Parietal Lobe and movement
The Parietal Lobe behind the Frontal Lobe in the middle top of the head is also responsible for movement activities, orientation, recognition, and perception. Damage in the back section of the Parietal lobe could contribute to balance and motor skills.

That Representative Giffords regained orientation, perception and recognition so quickly is in itself a miracle. However, damage in this section may be a part of her inability to move her right arm.

The Occipital Lobe and sight

The Occipital Lobe supports sight and interpretation of images. This indicates that the bullet inflicted injury in the left back area of the brain behind Representative Giffords' eye.

If there is less sight or the left eye is blind, there may be distortion or illusions of objects and persons in the opposite field. This might also lend itself to coordination or balance deficit issues.

Temporal Lobe and its vital functions

Reports state that Representative Giffords was struck in the top portion of the brain. It may be that the Temporal Lobe was spared entirely. This may be why she still has memory, can still function by following and making decisions on legislation and can hear and understand what she hears. She may never be quite the same, however, her ability to retrain her brain is reason to believe that her injury was confined above the more vital areas.

Brain Injury and Risk for Dementia

A new discovery reported in studies of traumatic brain injuries states that not all cases develop irreversible dementia. There is no evidence to prove risk of a single event. However, repeated mild concussions may increase risk of dementia diseases such as Alzheimer's. Other diseases, such as Parkinson's may occur from repeated injury to the brain. (Mohammed Ali, champion boxer) Parkinson's may or may not develop in the cognitive area of the brain.

Research and Development for Brain Injury

The vital and highly experienced health care professionals at the University Medical Center in Tucson and others that diagnosed and set up the recovery plan for Representative Gabrielle Giffords could not have acted so quickly if technology and research had not been available.

Support brain research and development by donation and/or urging congress to continue legislation for funds.

Online References

Brain Structures and Their Functions bryamaur.edu Serendip Studio
SingSurf.org Left Brain, Right Brain, Whole Brain?
CDDC Vermont Education -Occipital Lobe

University Medical Center Tucson AZ - reports of Gabrielle Giffords recovery
UA News.arizonaedu

NOTES

Summary
of Creating the Dynamic Dementia Care Team

Contents from "Caregiver Tips published at Examiner.com by Clarice Cook, September 28, 2010

According to the Alzheimer's Association of America, Alzheimer's is one of the most common causes of Dementia.

-People with Dementia do not necessarily have Alzheimer's

-Alzheimer's is not a normal symptom of aging.

Alzheimer's typically begins with short-term memory loss that lasts beyond the normal forgotten thought. In a normal situation, a person might rarely lose a line or topic in speech or forget the location of keys, etc.

There are common factors in onset dementia diseases such as Alzheimer's, in that recent memory loss is frequent. As the disease progresses for the Alzheimer's patient, long and short term memories fade away forever.

Symptoms in each person with a memory loss disease may progress differently from the onset. However, caregivers need to be aware and be ready to deal with many of the following issues for any person with brain injury or dementia.

Professional caregivers need to be alert to changes.

-Stay up to date and record changes.

-Be prepared to adjust to client's changing needs.

-Keep in close contact with care plan log and/or family or Client Care Coordinator to be aware of gradual changes.

-Research ways to cope with mood swings, changes in personality, increasing bouts of suspicion, withdrawal from communication, and lack of interest in beloved activities.

Find ways to alleviate stress over memory loss.

 -Clients may need constant reminders of medication times, appointments, and events.

 -Report when client shows frustration with financial or mental task (ex: checkbook).

 -Reassure client there will be help for forgotten task.

 -Do fun mental exercises approved by care plan.

 -Gently assist client to remember words and complete sentences.

 -Encourage verbalization about frustrations, anger, and sadness.

 -Empathize with client about feelings.

Communication with the client may become gradually more difficult. On every visit, realize Dementia and/or Alzheimer's clients may be confused with who and why there is someone else in the home.

-When entering the home, always make client aware early who you are.

-Check and avoid loud distractions and noises.

-Use a pleasant, not overly loud demeanor.

-Watch nonverbal body language (gestures, touch, and tone of voice).

-Smile and/or appropriately (but slowly) touch an arm or take a hand.

-Stay in front of client and slightly to the side out of reach of someone who regards you as a barrier or challenger.

-Make eye contact.

-Keep a pleasant voice, but loud enough for hearing impaired.

-Speak slowly, clearly and annunciate words.

-Never argue with a client.

-Keep questions and words simple and clear to client.

-If the client gets frustrated, have them talk out feelings.

-Stay with one subject or question at a time.

-Be patient and wait for answers.

-Keep sentences simple and emphasize key words.

-Give directions one-step at a time.

-Focus on past memories, childhood, and encourage conversations about positive family times and legacy.

In Retrospect: Caring for Persons with Dementia

Great caregivers, indeed certified and licensed health care professionals, have found themselves overwhelmed by clients/patients who are enduring the rigors of dementia. Caregivers and loved ones can better understand and care for the client/patient by researching self and being honest about their own very real passions and ambitions. Caring for self is a prerequisite of being an effective caregiver. Be real about expectations. Know goals are primarily monetary or primarily passion in life. It is important to know from deep within.

Care giving for persons with dementia, especially those with severe cases, is more intense and requires more from health care and in home ADL providers than is required for most care giving professions.

Through a basic knowledge of how the brain gathers, assimilates, and stores information and what happens when connections are broken, the caregiver and loved ones can find ways to alleviate the minute to minute challenges that the dementia patient faces.

By finding ways to replace broken links in communication, the effective caregiver can guide persons with memory loss through difficult times and buffer the connection between the client and loved ones. It is impossible for the damaged brain to understand reality. It is up to those around them to go to the world where that person lives. It is never effective to openly disagree or argue with the person with dementia. They are desperately clinging to dignity and self -worth and need to be validated.

Caregivers need to stay alert to changes and record them for health care professionals. Watch and be prepared to adjust to the ever-changing needs and moods of the client. Communicate with other caregivers and health care professionals to coordinate physical and mental health care.

Educate self and be open-minded to research by professionals and ideas of others knowledgeable in the field. Even scientist do not yet have all the answers, however, the experts, such as the Alzheimer's Association have come a long way in brain function, diseases and disorders. By researching reputable sites on the Internet, by experience and by learning about the person's needs, the caregiver can be extremely effective in helping the client and loved ones.

Be aware, watch body language, never argue with the client, and listen with an open mind. Learn how to cope with mood swings, changes in personality, increasing bouts of suspicion, withdrawal from communication, and loss of interest in previous activities.

Symptoms in each person with a memory loss disease may progress differently from the onset. However, caregivers need to be aware and be ready to deal with many of the following issues for any person with brain injury or dementia.

Find ways to alleviate stress over memory loss. Persons with memory loss may know about their diagnosis and this may be extremely stressful. There may not be a lot that the caregiver can do to stop the depression process, however, distractions may help for short periods.

Medication prescribed by medical providers may help to alleviate symptoms of depression, anxiety, and/or aggression. However, clients may need constant reminders to take their medications. According to the HIPPA rules for patients, clients have the right to refuse their meds. The only thing that a non-medical caregiver can do is to encourage and record the refusal if the attempt is unsuccessful.

Nutrition can make a big difference to alleviate symptoms, but never let mealtime become unpleasant. Present the meal with a home like and appetizing way with color (single colors with no design). If the client is overwhelmed by amounts of food, or too many selections, serve meals that please the client on large plates that make the portions seem small. Serve dessert separately. If the client does not eat a good meal, serve a supplemental drink and present it as "chocolate milk," a "shake," or "malt". If refusal is persistent, check for problems in the mouth or troubles swallowing. Foods that were normally enjoyed may no longer be pleasing. Try different foods. Notice if the client is starting to lose focus or needs increased assistance with silverware. Finger foods may be easier. Keep the place setting uncluttered.

The caregiver may be asked to drive to or remind the client about appointments or to shop. Patient rights also give the client the right to refuse. However, the caregiver can politely and gently encourage the afflicted person to do what is necessary for health care. Some things are not all that important, therefore, refusals should be reported to the client's power of attorney or other responsible person to make that decision.

Report when client shows frustration with financial or mental task (ex: checkbook). Offer reassurance of help if a client is upset about forgetting task. Encourage the client to verbalize frustrations, anger, and sadness and offer empathy. Then lead the client in calm conversation to a rational resolution or better outlook.

Follow the care plan closely and participate with the client on approved mental and physical exercises. Protect the client's self -esteem by gently assisting client in word games and completing sentences.

Communication with the client may become gradually more difficult. Symptoms of dementia are ever changing from minute to minute. With every visit and with every moment with the client, expect changes.

Scenario: The client has advanced to the point of not remembering people. Always make the client aware early on as to your identity, your presence, and that you are there to help them. Throughout a shift, the client may need reminders.

For instance: A client goes to the bathroom and then comes out and is surprised to see the caregiver. The caregiver should greet the client as though she or he just arrived. "Hello, I'm _____ (show your name on the badge) and I'm here to visit with you."

Check and avoid loud distractions and noises. Example: More than one electronic device going at the same time or too many people talking can create a confusing chaos. If there is a family gathering, make sure that the client is not overwhelmed.

Approach or interact with the client in calm and not over powering demeanor. Smile, keep a pleasant voice, and gauge the voice to the hearing level of the client. Sometimes caregivers speak too fast and overpower the client with unfamiliar words. Avoid slurring words, speak slowly, but not drawn out and exaggerated. The rule is to be clear, keep sentences short with annunciated words

Stay in front of the client, but be careful not to invade the client's space. This is especially important for the frustrated person. Watch body language, such as gestures, touch, and tone of voice, eye movement, and facial expression. Make eye contact in listening and speaking with clients. Be patient and wait for answers or to whatever they have to say.

Never argue or disagree with what the client has to say. Let them know that you heard what they had to say and then offer other suggestions, if necessary or if the statement is important. Always use the rule, "Pick the battles." However, never battle. Distract and use positive manipulation to keep the client safe. If the client is offering a general opinion, it is not important enough. Silent dismissal and distraction is in order.

Never take any comment as personal. Remember that the client is unaware that they are being rude or hateful.

Give directions or suggestions one-step at a time. Keep it simple, but not childlike. Remember that the client is an adult.

In conversing with the client, focus on past memories, childhood, and encourage conversations about positive family times and legacy. However, if the client has dementia, asking the question, "Do you remember?" is counterproductive in most cases. To interact with the dementia client about the past, it might be appropriate to show them scrapbooks or pictures and wait for them to tell you their stories. The key words are "their stories." If the caregiver (family or professional) knows that the stories or identification of persons is inaccurate, it is best to let it pass. It is not important that facts are straight. It is imperative that the client is happy.

Adhere to the rules of HIPPA. It is the law and violators can be prosecuted. Never restrain a violent or aggressive client or loved one. If a situation has escalated, stand a distance away or exit the area after ensuring that the client is safe and call for help. That may be to call 911, the power of attorney or other authority, whoever is listed on the care plan.

Take care of yourself, keep the client safe, stay calm, patient and positive, engage the client in happy interaction or let them have privacy, learn to read body language, go with the flow, stay in front of them in conversation, give the client space, make eye contact, listen with an open mind, never argue, respect the clients dignity, never take client comments personal, follow the care plan, record incidents and important information, give medication reminders...never administer meds, unless authorized, allow refusal and record it, encourage nutrition, but allow refusal, strictly adhere to the rules of HIPPA.

There will be times when the caregiver will make mistakes. Mistakes are lessons learned and opportunities to improve. Take time to note the lesson and continue.

The best caregivers have an open mind and an open heart. Never close the mind or heart, but remember to save respect for self.

Feel free to take time to take the following self-test. Be perfectly honest. There are no wrong or right answers. The tests are merely to help persons analyze themselves and make decisions about care giving as a possible career or as a family member.

Assessing Self Values in the role of the Caregiver

There is no doubt a huge requirement for loving our persons that we care for. I have heard it said, "All they need is love." However, within that love lies facing the truth about how a care person faces the challenges, what talents they possess, the limits to which they can sacrifice time, emotion, physical and mental stamina and what role they can take in caring for a family member or client.

There is no shame in being truthful and honestly taking a lesser or stronger role, depending on circumstances and ability. Being respectful of others involved and letting the "puzzle" fit naturally can avoid caregiver burnout and allow each member of a team to enjoy a loved one and allow for quality of life for the person afflicted with memory loss.

Each family member wants to be validated. The best thing that a family can do is to learn to give a little and accept their part equally with respect...idealistically. Getting everyone on board with that is difficult.

Persons with dementia will exhibit more strongly those traits that are dominate throughout their life in most cases that I've worked with.

Dawson was always a proud man and bragged incessantly. He grew angry sometimes to the point of having a temper tantrum when people disagreed with him. Yet, he would get worked up and say, "People who know it all just set me off. For him, it was the people with a different viewpoint who were the pompous and arrogant ones. His logic is his own.

Gabriel has served in many wars, was successful at winning in sports and all aspects of his life, including business. He's 95 and a millionaire, now with diagnosed Alzheimer's. His wife and he have had an extremely volatile relationship for 65 years. She's eighty-six and still fairly sharp. Her forgetfulness is most likely due to stress. Gabriel verbally attacks his wife with every waking moment for what he considers to be sloppy and unorganized housekeeping and life decisions. He tells everyone that it is his wife that has dementia, not he. When the dementia practitioners explain that Gabriel's behavior is due to the disease, the wife rejects that saying that, "He's always been that way. I've had to endure that for fifty-five years. The practitioner asks, "Has it always been as severe as it has been since he's home most of the time?" She admits that it has gotten worse. Indeed, Gabriel had to be taken to the mental health facility by the police because of his attack on his wife.

It is the disease that brings out the worst because in the frontal lobe where control and logic reside, the neurons and transmitters are so damaged that the brain can no longer sort out the feelings from the amygdala in the center hippocampus and put what is being seen, heard, felt, and tasted together into a logical understanding.

NOTES

Self-Test -The Process

Draw a line down the middle of a blank page. On one column write down who you think, you are according to the following list. On the other column write down the words that describe how you think, others think of you. This exercise is for your eyes only. Show it to no one. Be perfectly honest.

After taking the complete sessions for care giving, look at your list and decide where you fit into a family team or as a professional caregiver. Be honest with yourself in order to be able to survive the journey that you/your family/your loved one/your clients are facing and prevent stress and turmoil that could otherwise result.

Refer back to the information in this manual in making your assessment and coming to the conclusion. Some questions apply to mainly to professionals; however, all can be considered one way or the other by all caregivers, depending upon the circumstances.

The goal is to find out whether:

Do you stay within abilities?

Do you challenge yourself?

Can you take supervision without complaint?

Do you plan your life or do you fall into events and decisions?

Do you have goals or is life just one day after another?

Is your goal in the health field or are you just remaining where you are in order to pay the bills for other goals for what your dream really is?

Are you working in your dream field or are you just working to pay the bills?

Do you work to live or live to work?

When dealing with a difficult client, do you feel empathetic?

Do you feel confident or intimidated when faced with an angry, sad, or unresponsive person?

Are you able to work alone?

Are you loyal?

Can you accept that life will slow down, and it means taking each minute at a time?

Can you accept that sometimes, some things are just not that important?

Do you,

Make time to unwind and use positive ways to handle stress?

Fear other persons in time of temper outburst?

Feel like giving up on a regular basis?

Have common sense in stress or other situations?

Think before action?

Have vision about results of actions?

Have a love of humanity?

Respect and value honor?

Want to be wealthy?

Value wisdom?

Enjoy working with others?

Seek meaningful work?

Encourage and try to have a positive attitude?

Respect order...stability, conformity?

Acknowledge mistakes and seek ways to resolve resulting problems?

Give others credit for their strengths?

Forgive other weaknesses?

What is important to you?

Personal development

Security

Fast-paced work

Financial gain

Freedom of life choices

Growth of self

Family

Helping other people

Honesty

Independence

Influencing others

Inner harmony

Pleasure

Power and authority

Privacy

Public service

Purity

Quality

Quality relationships

Recognition and respect

Reputation

Responsibility/accountability

Integrity

Intellectual status

Involvement

Job tranquility

Knowledge

Leadership

Location

Loving what you do

Change and variety

Close relationships

Community

Competence

Competition

Cooperation

Country

Creativity

Decisiveness

Democracy

Ecological awareness

Economic security

Effectiveness

Ethical practice

Excellence

Excitement

Exercise

Expertise

Fame

Fast living

Achievement

Advancement

Affection

Arts

Challenging problems

Change and variety

Quality time management

Your values are not your values unless you live them. Will the values you have chosen work in a health care environment?

Are you?

Forward thinking

Idling

Able to help clients unwind and de-escalate stress, tension, and anger

Pompous

Able to put self-welfare of others ahead of self,

Able to sacrifice self-needs when necessary for others

Able to value self-worth

Trustworthy

Honest

"White Liar"

Dishonestly Manipulative

Positive Manipulator

Judgmental

Non-Judgmental

Reliable

Procrastinator

Responsible

Perceptive

Trustworthy

Goal oriented

Thoughtful

Good problem solver

Passionate about caring for other

Health conscious

Self-respect

Serene

Sophisticated

Stable

Want status

Able to supervise

Value integrity

Acknowledge weaknesses

Recognize strengths

Compassionate

Patient

Honorable in the face of criticism

Make the most of constructive criticism

Empathetic and able to stay calm when someone is upset and yelling at you.

Honest, appreciate and seek truth

Nature lover

Open and honest and being with open and honest people

Up for physical challenge

Able to work with diversity

Able to deal with crisis

Do your choices of talents and abilities fit a dementia care field of employment?

The Family Caregiver- Team Building

The following is not always done by family members, because there may not be that many persons available for these tasks. Sometimes, only one person is responsible. However, if there are enough family members, it is good to have a team to help with caring for another adult, especially one with dementia issues.

Your Talents

The Organizer, Business minded: I am organized, able to negotiate, find information to present to the team with regard to insurance companies, Medicare, hospitals, care teams, facilities, help organizations, equipment companies, legal issues, etc.
The Bookkeeper: I am the banker. I am able to keep track of funds and keep records of how the money has been spent to present a financial report to the team.

In Home Care

The Housekeeper and Maintenance Person: I am the organized person who can either physically make sure that the home is kept clean and safe or orchestrate others to do the maintenance and care of the home. I research companies to make sure that my elder person does not fall victim to fraud or elder abuse at the hands of unscrupulous home maintenance persons.

The In-Home Caregiver

As the person responsible for the actual physical care or director of physical care of someone who cannot care for themselves, I am most in need of soul searching to make sure that I am mentally and physically able to withstand the long, goodbye journey. I am trained to assist the client or family member with activities of daily living, including nutrition, medical administration and monitoring, maintaining a clean environment, etc. This may also include bathing, dealing with incontinence, ambulation, and many other duties that a Certified Nurse Aide is trained to do.

In the case of a person with Alzheimer's and some other dementias, additional skills are needed in dealing with someone with problem behavior issues. The caregiver must be adept in interacting, corresponding, encouraging appropriate activities, and distracting a person with neurological pathway damage.

The caregiver must realize that every person is different, since there are no two people on earth who are exactly the same. The damage in the brain is different for every person. Reactions and symptoms are likely to be different from one minute to the next. Keeping expectations reasonable, being able to adapt and flexible to change is important for success in taking care of a person with dementia.

Team respect, love, understanding, and tolerance

For families, Alzheimer's in particular is one of the most difficult and heartbreaking of all diseases. Losing a parent or loved one in a long goodbye can break the bonds of the strongest of families. It is extremely important that the entire team support each other with respect, love, understanding, and tolerance. If one team member seems to be faltering, respectfully find out how other team members can fill in the gap. Remember that no one is perfect, everyone is doing the best possible, and as Harry Truman once said, "It is amazing what you can accomplish if you do not care who gets the credit."

Comment [CC]:

NOTES

Recommended Reading at Examiner.com
Some of the content of this manual is from the online at examiner.com caregiver in Grand Rapids Clarice Cook or at examiner.com caregiver in national Clarice Cook

Suggested Online Reading
Clarice Cook is the author of caregiving articles at Examiner.com. Among the articles are the following for suggested reading.

-Health Care Team: Intervention for Spousal Caregivers to Prevent Elder Abuse

-Caregiver Tips: Bed Ridden Patients - positioning-and-changing-linens

-Caregiver Tips: Safety Equipment for Elderly and Disabled Clients

-Caregiver Training Tips for Safe Ambulation to Avoid Bone Fracture

-Laughter Therapy and Benefits for Cancer Patients and Survivors

Creating the Dynamic Dementia Care Team is a prelude to Memory Path Care Solutions. Both manuals are authored by Clarice Cagle Cook and available for Audible Narrated and Produced at ACX.com

Other books by Clarice Cagle Cook
Fiction
Legacy from the Wake Journals
Echo from Shady Mountain
Justice for Echo Valley
Non-Fiction
Memory Path Care Solutions

Thank you for reading. Both positive and negative reviews are welcome. Find review opportunity at online bookstores or write to me at creatorwriting@outlook.com. or message at www.facebook.com/cccwriter.

www.ingramcontent.com/pod-product-compliance
Lightning Source LLC
Chambersburg PA
CBHW081501170526
45166CB00008B/2509